Hair Care Rehab

The Ultimate Hair Repair & Reconditioning Manual

Hair Care Rehab

The Ultimate Hair Repair & Reconditioning Manual

Audrey Davis-Sivasothy

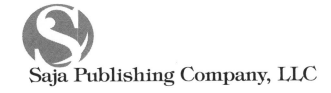

Saja Publishing Company, LLC

Printed in the United States of America.
Cover and Interior Design by Velin Saramov

Publisher's Cataloging-in-Publication Data

Davis-Sivasothy, Audrey
Hair care rehab: the ultimate hair repair & reconditioning manual/ Audrey Davis-Sivasothy.
p. cm.
Includes index.
ISBN-978-0-9845184-5-6 (paperback)
ISBN-978-0-9845184-6-9 (electronic)

I. Hair—Care and hygiene. Title.
2012901957
First Edition

To all of us—

Because we *all* have some kind of hair drama.

Contents

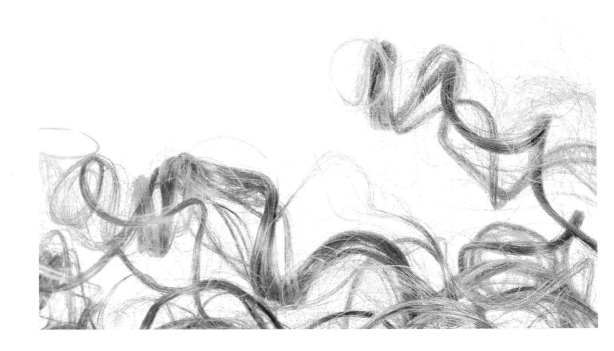

Unit I:
The Intervention

n. in-ter-ven-shuhn

a frank meeting or confrontation with addicts about their behavior and its consequences by friends, family members and others who care about them

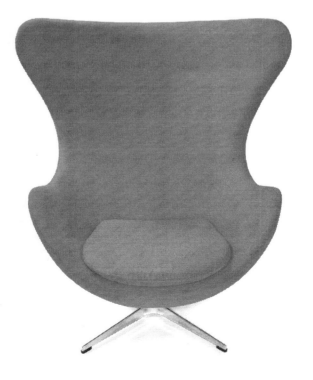

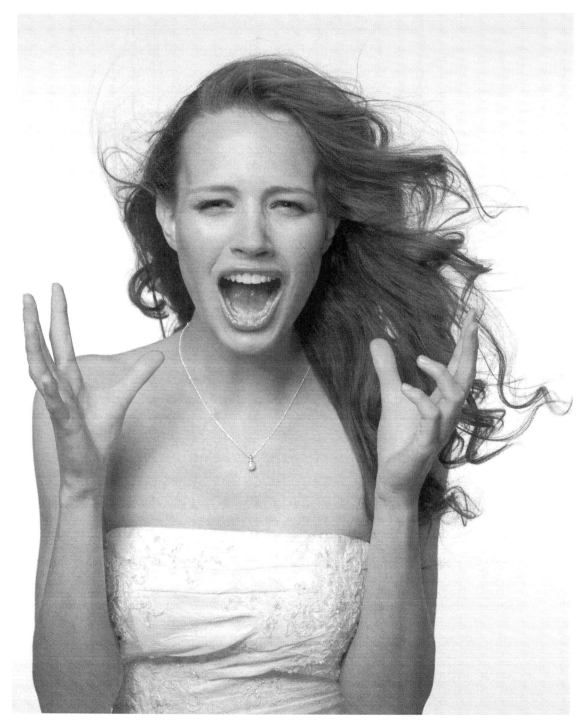

Figure 1 - Is your hair driving you insane? Maybe it's time for a little rehab.

Having a Bad Hair Day Life?

The relationship we have with our hair is just like any other long-term relationship in life. Right? There are those rare, magical moments when everything is right and simply falls into place—and then there are those long, epic battles that try the hearts and souls of men (and women!). Chances are, you're reading this book because those rare, magical moments are—well, *rare*. You emerge from the bathroom each morning having fought the battle of your life with dry, breaking hair—uncontrollably limp and oily hair—or frizzy, erratically shedding hair. Or maybe that battle is not with your hair at all, but with an itchy, dry scalp that is inconveniently buried under layers of white flakes. Whatever the case, you're desperately looking for an exit strategy, FAST!

Hair drama affects us all—whether your hair is thick, fine, stick-straight, wavy, coily, or curly! Fortunately for you, you've found the road to recovery.

Welcome to *Hair Care Rehab*. This is your hair care intervention.

Now, before you say, **What's the big deal? It's just hair**—stop yourself and think about it for a moment.

How often do people describe us by the way our hair looks?
You know, the girl with the shiny, brown hair . . .frizzy curls . . .retro bangs . . . gorgeous, long layers, etc.

How often are we judged by it?

Paula has really let herself go. Her grays are taking over.

And what other personal feature has the power to completely ruin a date—a wedding—your confidence—like hair?

Nothing.

Let's face it: Hair is important. You are holding this book because hair is important! And if your hair is in questionable shape, this is your wakeup call! This book is here to whip you into shape. It's not going to waste your valuable time with the typical useless fluff—although we totally promise not to bore you! Honestly, there are already tons of books, magazines, and Internet blogs out there if you want the mindless fluff scattered about and have time to sift through and filter it all. But, if you want *rehab* . . . if you want *solutions* and *results* for a variety of common hair issues—this is your step-by-step manual for a better hair future. For some of you, it won't be easy—but if you take your rehab one step and one day at a time, we're pretty sure you'll come to a happier hair place.

Sound good? Well, let's go!

It's Not You, It's Me

We're all borderline obsessed with our hair, and by most accounts, it starts somewhere in junior high school. Our hair becomes our latest fashion experiment—and we do some pretty incredible things to it in the name of beauty. We continue the drama on into our adult years and, well, between our hectic, high-heat, multi–color-shifting styling routines and our less-than-perfect dietary regimens (anyone else have a love affair with the microwave?), how does our hair or scalp ever stand a chance?

We go to amazing lengths to control our hair—and although it may seem to work for a time, we usually end up with fried straw when it's all said and done. If every day is a fight (and it's one that you are definitely not winning), it's time to face the enemy head on. Unfortunately, almost 99 percent of the time, we are the enemy. We are abusers! (The old cliché *"It's not you, it's me"* really comes into play when we are looking at hair damage.)

But that's no earth-shattering revelation, is it?

You knew your hair-frying and dyeing escapades would eventually catch up with you! Although your haircare "drug of choice" and level of addiction may not be the same as the next person's, the bottom line is that you are the common denominator in this hair destruction equation. The change has to start with you, and that's true for any relationship!

In this book, we'll take you through three phases of rehab: Intervention, Detox and Hair Therapy.

In the *Intervention* phase, you'll learn the basics about your hair and its structure. You'll also learn about the four healthy-hair killers and how to work around (or with) these hair care drugs of choice.

In *Detox*, you will discover our Five-Step strategy for hair repair and ways to fight back against damage.

In *Hair Therapy*, the final phase, you will find a wealth of simple traditional and nontraditional therapies to help you alleviate common problems such as dandruff, psoriasis, hair breakage, and porous hair. You'll even find a host of treatments that you can make at home to fit your budget. What are you waiting for? Let's go!

Figure 2- Most hair care issues are caused by the demands we place on our hair.

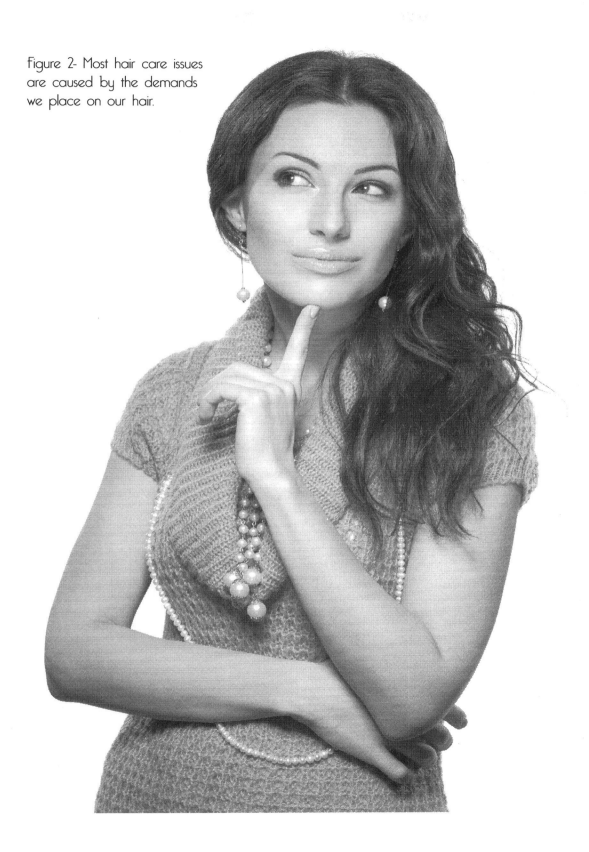

Chapter 1:

Let's Start Off with What Is Not True

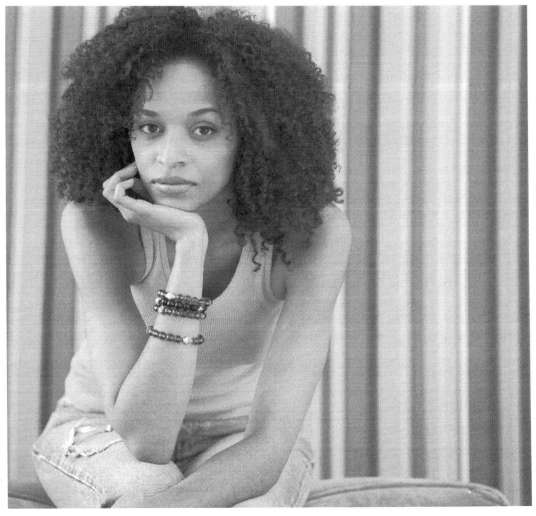

Figure 3- There are so many myths in hair care that it can be difficult to filter out the noise.

I n our quest for healthier hair, we are certain to come across myths, stereotypes, and, well, just flat-out bad ideas. Before we start rehab, let's start off with what is simply not true. It's hard to imagine how some of the ideas floating around still manage to see the light of day, but are we really surprised? The world's share of hair care gurus, world-renowned stylists, multi–billion-dollar product companies, and even dear Aunt Gretchen—keep many of the old wives' tales alive and well. Seasoned hair care veterans can spot the top offenders from a mile away, but those who are new to hair care may have trouble separating fact from fiction.

Let's take a quick look at seven bad hair care ideas that just won't die:

1. There are magic pills (or oils, serums, balms) to grow our hair faster, stronger, or thicker.

Unfortunately, no. Hair growth is genetically predetermined and controlled by our hormones. Unless a pill or product can affect our genes or hormones, there's no hope that it might grow our hair. (This includes prenatal vitamins, too. You can blame the upsurge in hormone levels during pregnancy for those vibrant tresses!) Basic vitamin supplements can offer slight improvements in our hair's quality, *but only if* our body truly lacks the particular vitamin or mineral being taken. If you are healthy and your diet is fairly balanced, your body will simply flush out the excess supplements you give it.

2. Trimming will make your hair grow stronger, longer, faster, or thicker.

Since hair is dead, cutting the ends has no effect on what happens at the scalp level. Strands will grow at the same predetermined rate each month, and individual strands will grow in at the same thickness as before. While trimming or cutting

the hair does *seem* to give the appearance of thicker hair at first, this is only because all of the freshly trimmed hairs now have the same, clear endpoint. Hair that was fine or thin before will start to appear fine or thin again once it grows out. This is because older hairs are constantly being replaced by shorter, newer hairs, and faster-growing hairs continue to grow in at their rapid pace.

3. Expensive products do more!

Not necessarily. You should always look for ingredients over brand names. There are just as many poorly formulated high-end products as there are bargain ones—and just as many worthy expensive products as there are bargain ones too! Spending more on your hair care won't hurt you (well, maybe your pocketbook and your pride), but do not immediately dismiss the economy brands. They may be a better deal for you.

4. Products made for or marketed to (insert race/ethnicity) cannot be used by those of other backgrounds.

False! The ingredients in a product matter much more than who the product is marketed to. In fact, most products have the same set of three to five base ingredients! Products for "ethnic" hair types tend to be more moisturizing and have more oils and proteins than products for other hair types. But damaged hair needs a good dose of moisture, proteins, and oil to regain its healthy appearance. The same holds true for products marketed to those with color-treated hair. Even if your hair is not colored, using a product for color-treated hair can still be beneficial because these shampoo formulas tend to be gentler (to preserve easily washed away hair color) and conditioners tend to be super-conditioning, but lightweight to help reduce dryness from the coloring process.

5. **Hair can be repaired—permanently—with a conditioner or repair product.**

We will get into this more in Chapter 3, but the answer to this, sadly, is also no. Hair can be repaired (patched up) only temporarily through regular conditioning that can smooth down the outer layers of the hair shaft and give the appearance of healthier hair. A good conditioner can also prevent damage from occurring in the first place. We'll show you how to do this in the upcoming pages.

6. **Washing your hair too often leads to dryness.**

This depends. Hair can be cleansed as often as you like without dryness, provided you use the proper products to retain moisture. Those who generally have naturally drier hair types (i.e., those of us with curls and highly textured hair) often shy away from frequent cleansing—but water is not the enemy! It's the stripping shampoos and mediocre conditioners we use that are to blame for dryness. Using the proper moisturizing and conditioning products at wash time will actually increase your hair's hydration.

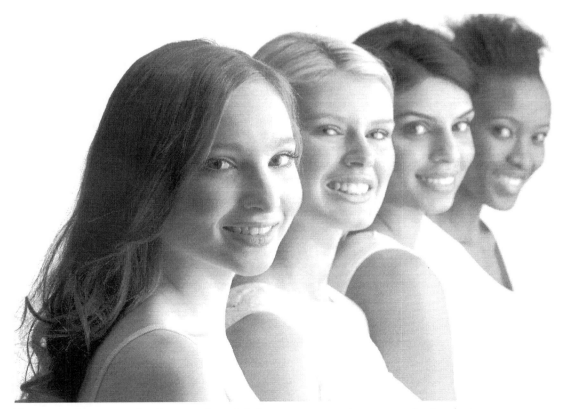

Figure 4- Airing out the hair myths will help you in your journey to better hair.

7. Hair can "get used to" hair products and brands.

Has it ever felt like your favorite shampoo or conditioner product just stopped working? You may have heard that you need to rotate your products every once in awhile so that your hair does not get "tired of" or "used to" your staples. Not true! Our hair doesn't get used to certain brands; what happens is that certain products (usually conditioners, serums and oils) tend to leave behind mild residue that turns into product buildup on your hair. This buildup can make it seem like your old products just aren't doing their jobs anymore. When buildup occurs, it usually also means that your shampoo is too mild to remove the conditioner/oil layer during your cleansing phase. Switching to a stronger, clarifying shampoo once or twice a month to clear up any product buildup often does the trick.

Chapter 2:

Hair & Scalp: Just the Basics

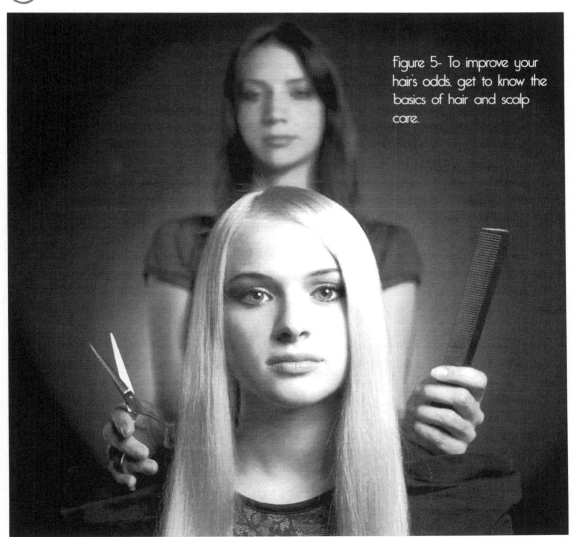

figure 5- To improve your hair's odds, get to know the basics of hair and scalp care.

We demand a lot of our hair. Seriously! Many of us ask our hair to do things Mother Nature never intended. While our hair is a really strong, resilient fiber, it is not immune to stress and damage. Dryness and breakage can creep up on us, and hair thinning can occur over time. In order to understand hair damage, it is important to have a basic understanding of hair structure. Now, before you start yawning and flipping through pages—don't worry! We'll try to drive home key points quickly without bogging you down with the details! Hair science can admittedly get a little—well—boring. *Visine, anyone?*

So, let's take a step back and cover just the basics:

Hair: Just the Basics!

Every new hair starts growing from one of more than 100,000 *follicles* deep within the skin. The number of hair follicles we have is determined by genetics and also, interestingly, by our hair color. We are born with as many follicles as we'll ever have. The base of the hair follicle is also known as the *hair bulb*. The cells in the hair bulb, fed by an intricate network of capillaries, divide every one to three days—a rate of cell division that makes them some of the fastest-reproducing cells in the human body. As the cells harden, they are packed together and forced up through the scalp. These hardened, packed-together cells are the long threads of hair that we see. Once the hair leaves the follicle, it is no longer living tissue. This means that it can be cut and styled without causing you pain.

The *oil (sebaceous)* glands are part of the hair follicle. These glands produce oil (sebum) at the rate of about an ounce every one hundred days to condition and lubricate the hair fiber. If your hair is oily, you are probably quite familiar with these glands!

The Shaft

A basic hair shaft is comprised of two (sometimes three) layers: the outer cuticle, the cortex, and (occasionally) the medulla. You will hear a lot about the outer cuticle throughout this book—it's really that important.

Cuticle

The cuticle layer determines whether or not our hair actually *looks* healthy. It's our hair's first line of defense against breakage. Think of it as armor for your strands, protecting your hair from you and the rest of the outside world! The cuticle's job is to keep precious moisture contained inside the hair strand and to ward off wear and tear from the environment. Under a microscope, the cuticle's scales overlap and look like shingles on a roof. Processes such as coloring, perming, brushing, washing, and styling damage these protective scales and cause them to chip and lift up over time.

Without a doubt, the healthy appearance of hair depends almost entirely upon the condition of the cuticle. Lifted cuticle scales mean dry, unruly hair. Tattered cuticles reflect light poorly, and increased friction between raised cuticle scales on multiple strands prevents hair from moving well when styled. Dullness and lack of movement are key signs of hair damage.

Did you know that no matter how well we take care of our hair, it always goes from *bad to worse* as we move from root to tip along the fiber? This is especially true if the hair happens to be fairly long. Cuticle damage is concentrated along the mid-shaft and ends simply because *long hair is old hair.* The hair along the ends has been around longer than hair near the scalp, and so it's been washed, ironed, blown dry, and braided more than the hair at the top of the strand. It is not uncommon for cuticle degradation at the very tip of the hair shaft to be so complete that the inner hair layers are completely exposed. Because it is easily accessible, the cuticle is the layer that most hair treatments work on. *Hair Care Rehab* will give you handy advice for protecting this layer of the hair fiber!

Cortex

Fiercely guarded by layers and layers of cuticle, the cortex is perhaps the single most important layer of hair. While the cuticle determines whether our hair actually looks healthy, our hair gets its basic character—its color, texture, strength, and elasticity (stretchiness) from the cortex. (In fact, the hair's outer cuticle layer is colorless—the hair color we see is the color of the inner cortex!) For those with fine to medium hair strands (hair strands that are less than the thickness of a typical sewing thread), the cortex is the innermost portion of the hair shaft. If you cut a hair strand in half and look at it through a microscope, you'd see that the cortex makes up the greatest part of the hair fiber, accounting for 80 to 90 percent of the strand's total weight.

The Medulla

The medulla is found at the core of the hair shaft only in those with thick or coarse hair. Those

with naturally blonde hair, or fine hair, usually lack a medulla. To date, scientists have not yet determined the medulla's real purpose or its role in hair care. We won't deal with it here, but for kicks, it's good to know that it may be there.

Hair Texture & Type

When we work with our natural hair textures and types, we always end up with the healthiest hair. That's just a hair law! Big problems only come in when we try to change or work against what nature has given us: trying to make fine hair look thicker, curly hair look straighter, or raven-colored hair look lighter, for example.

Knowing your hair's texture and type will help you determine which kinds of products you'll need to use, how much heat styling you can bear, or how much handling you can tolerate while still keeping your hair looking great. In this section, we'll run you through the following:

- Hair Textures: Fine, Medium, Thick/Coarse
- Hair Shapes/Types: Straight, Wavy, Curly, Kinky-Curly/Coily

Hair Texture

Regardless of whether your hair is straight, wavy, or super curly, the three basic hair textures we have are *fine, medium and thick/coarse.* Now, you would *think* that "texture" would describe how the hair actually feels to the touch (soft, silky, rough, etc.) or even how much hair there is on the head. But, unfortunately, I don't make the rules here! Texture does not describe how the hair feels or how much hair you actually have on your scalp. Instead, each one of the three hair textures refers to the *thickness of the individual strands of hair* you have, usually when compared to a basic sewing thread. Fine strands are usually thinner than a thread, *medium strands* are about the same width or slightly thinner than a thread, and thick strands are usually the same

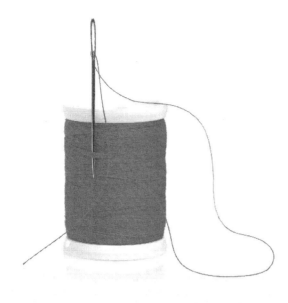

Figure 6- A sewing thread can help you determine your hair's texture.

width or thicker than a thread. You may have *fine strands* but lots and lots of them, making it appear that you have thick, full hair. Or you may have thick individual strands, but only a few of them, making it appear that your hair is quite thin. Coarse hair, by the same token, is not rough hair; it's hair that has thick, strong strands.

How can you determine whether your hair strands are fine, medium, or thick/coarse? If simple thread comparisons don't cut it, try this test:

1. **Take a single shed hair from your comb or brush and lay it on a sheet of white paper.**

- If your hair is medium, you'll see it easily against the paper, but it won't feel stiff or wiry.
- If your hair is fine, it will be barely visible against the paper and will be hard to grasp with your fingers.
- If your hair is thick/coarse, it will stand out clearly against the white paper and

will feel strong, stiff, and wiry in your hands.

2. **Part your hair down the center.**

- If your hair is fine, your part may appear "scalpy," or your hair may not give good coverage of the scalp outside of the parting.
- If your hair is either medium or thick/coarse, you will see very little or no scalp outside of the parting.

Keep in mind that your hair texture also has very little to do with the actual shape of your hair fiber. For example, your hair type may be straight or curly and still be a fine, medium, or thick/coarse texture. Also note that hair textures may vary on different parts of your head.

NOTE: There is a difference between the terms *hair texture* and *textured hair*. In cosmetology, *hair texture* refers to the width of an individual strand— but textured hair refers to the large class of curly, tightly coiled, spiraled and kinky hair types in general. It's possible to have *textured hair* (curly, coily hair) with a medium hair texture (strand thickness), for example.

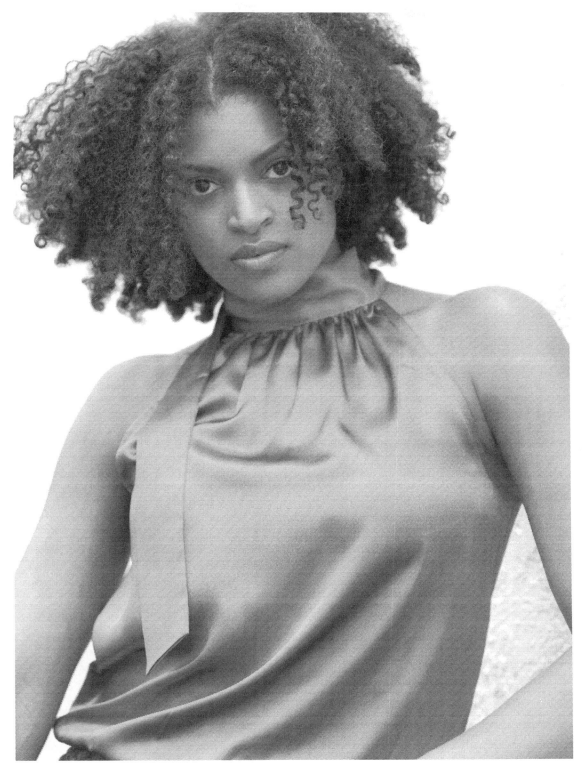

Figure 7- *Hair texture* refers to strand thickness, while *textured hair* refers to curly, kinky and tightly coiled hair.

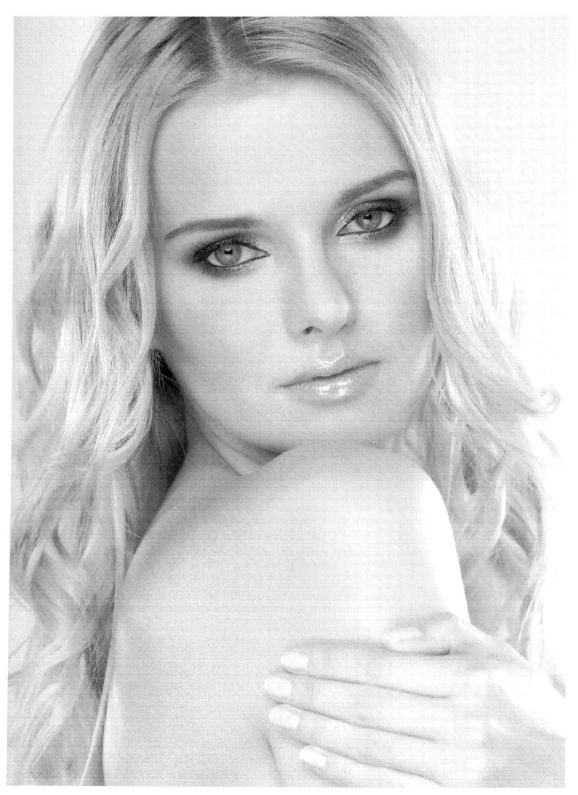

Figure 8- Fine hair has the smallest diameter and is the most fragile.

Fine Hair

Fine hair strands tend to be the most delicate and the easiest to damage and break. These fragile hairs are often very light to the touch and tend to fall flat against the head, no matter how much volumizing and teasing work is done! Interestingly, those with fine hair tend to have the *most* hair strands, since more hair strands are needed to cover the same scalp area as thicker strands. That's probably a surprise to those with fine hair who fight for volume! Having more strands per square inch also means that naturally fine hair tends to be oilier than other hair types since each hair comes equipped with its own oil gland.

Fine hair is very flexible, but it really has to fight hard to hold a style. This type of hair usually has only two of the three possible hair layers: just a cortex and a protective cuticle.

Naturally straight fine hair is glossy when it hasn't been damaged by chemicals or the environment. Curly girls can have fine hair too, although the hair's overall "bigness" can make it seem otherwise. Fine-stranded curlies tend to have fragile, baby-soft tresses that often feel weightless. If the hair is kinky/tightly curled and fine, it should be handled with the greatest care.

Fine hair is often mistaken for *thin hair*. Remember, the word fine refers to strand size. The word *thin* refers to scalp coverage. When fine hair is combined with thin scalp coverage, it can be really distressing, especially if the hair was fuller before. This is usually what happens as we age: Beginning in our late thirties to early forties, our scalps simply produce finer and finer individual strands. Eventually, some follicles stop producing hair altogether, resulting in less scalp coverage or balding.

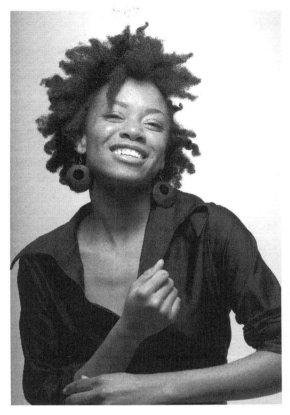

Figure 9- Textured hair can also be made up of fine strands.

Blondes tend to have the finest hair strands, but they outdo brunettes, redheads, and raven-colored hair types in the sheer number of strands that they have.

Medium Hair

Medium hair, the most common type, is neither thick nor fine. Together, the strands aren't feather light and airy, nor are they heavy and draping. Medium strands provide good coverage of the scalp, whether the hair is wet or dry.

When medium-textured hair is healthy, it tends to hold styles quite well without falling flat. Medium hairs have two of the three possible hair layers (cortex and protective cuticle) and may contain bits of the third inner layer (medulla) if the strands are closer to the thick side.

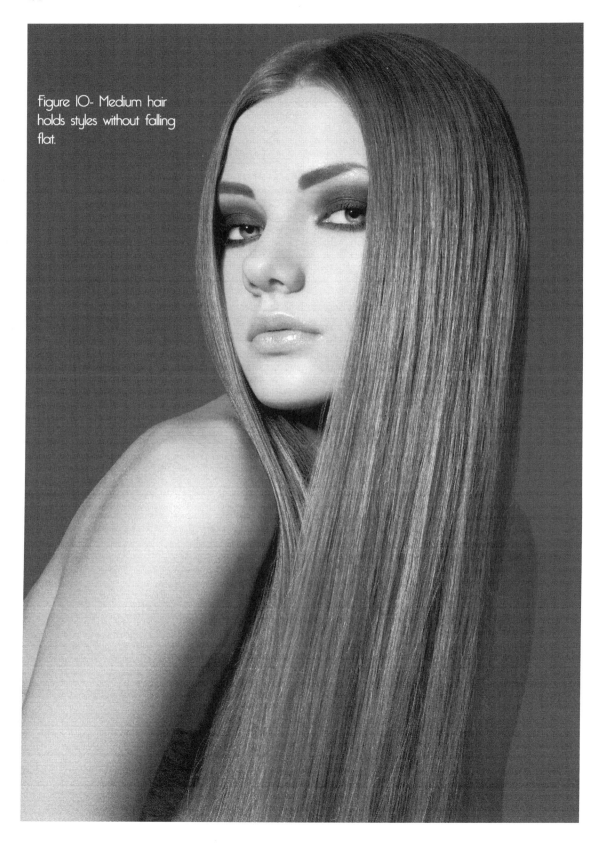

Figure 10- Medium hair holds styles without falling flat.

Thick/Coarse Hair

Thick hair strands are usually strong and quite wiry because they contain all three layers of hair (medulla, cortex, and cuticle). In fact, the thicker the strands are, the more rigid they will be. Thick strands give the scalp good coverage, and you can rarely see through to the scalp unless the hair is parted.

Often also referred to as "coarse" hair, this hair usually takes longer to dry than other hair textures and can be resistant to coloring and other chemical treatments. One benefit of coarse hair is that it is extremely heat tolerant and breakage-resistant, meaning that it can handle quite a bit more torture (and still look gorgeous) than other hair types. Because it is the most durable hair on earth, most human hair weaves are made from this type of hair. Lucky girls!

Hair Shape/Type

In addition to classifying our hair by texture, we can also classify it according to the actual shape of the hair fiber: straight, wavy, curly, and kinky-curly/coily. To determine your hair shape and type, it's best to work with freshly washed and air-dried hair with no products added. Hair should be rinsed in cold water quickly as a final rinse prior to allowing it to dry naturally.

Straight Hair

Naturally straight hair is the strongest, most resilient of all hair types and has a glossy, high-octane shine when it is healthy. Why is straight hair so shiny? It simply reflects light back to the eye better than any other hair type. If the hair is damaged, however, shine will be considerably reduced. Straight hair usually resists attempts to curl it and can be oily at times because natural oil from the scalp spreads through straight hairs faster than through other hair types. Wavy and curly girls who crave straight locks often go to some pretty interesting lengths to get there;

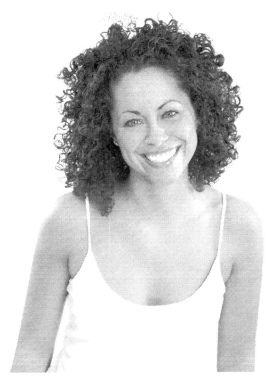

Figure 11- Curly hair can also be medium textured, although the shape of the hair may make it appear thicker.

unfortunately, this can be really hard on curly hair over time and always damages it in the process. In fact, going from curly to straight too often can cause curly girls to lose their curls almost entirely.

Wavy Hair

Wavy hair is often considered to be straight or curly hair with an attitude—and for good reason! Achieving the perfect waves can be a balancing act between frizziness and lankness on any given day! Although wave definition varies from person to person, and even on the same head, waves tend to form predictable cascading S-shapes along their length. Wavy hair usually lies very flat on the top of the head near the roots and gains its wavy character midway down and through to the ends of the hair. For this reason, there are millions of straight-haired folks with

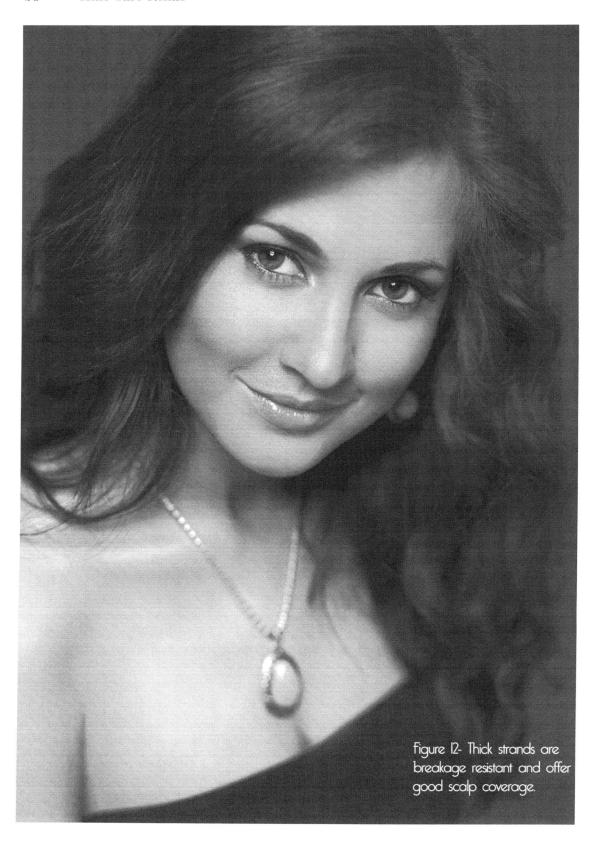

Figure 12- Thick strands are breakage resistant and offer good scalp coverage.

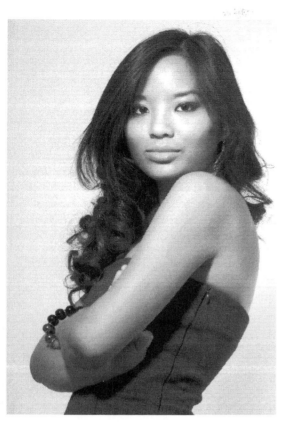

Figure 13- Thick strands have higher heat tolerance than other hair types.

short hair who are really wavy-haired folks or even curlies; their hair just hasn't reached the length to prove it! Healthy wavy hair curls and straightens with ease, and humidity tends to bring out the waves.

Curly Hair

Perhaps the greatest range of hair-strand shapes exists in the curly hair category, in which curls can be as large as beer cans or as small as coffee stirrers. Curly hair can appear extremely thick when you take in the big picture, but separating out a few curls often reveals that the strands themselves are actually quite fine—especially for the larger-diameter curl types. The larger the curls are, the shinier they will naturally appear. The curliest hair types tend to have more sheen (matte shine) than true shine.

What are the top three issues that most curly girls face? Frizz, lack of curl definition, and shrinkage! Frizz is just a natural part of being curly—although it's less of a problem for some than for others. Curl definition is best when hair is healthy, hasn't been fought with heat, is superhydrated, and is styled with the correct products and techniques to achieve the desired look. While some curl types shrink less than others, the coiliest curls can shrink more than 50 to 75 percent of their actual length!

For a great introduction to curly hair care, I recommend picking up a copy of Lorraine Massey's *Curly Girl: The Handbook*. From tightly coiled zigzag to corkscrew, Botticelli, and what she calls S'wavy, Massey breaks down curl care to a science.

Kinky-Curly/Coily (Textured Hair)

The tightest of curly strands can be classified as kinky-curly, coily or simply, textured. Textured hair strands can range from very fine to wiry/coarse, but what makes this hair unique is the wide variety of O-, S-, and Z-shaped curl patterns, which can exist in any combination on a single head and even along a single strand! Like curly hair, kinky-curly strands are also densely packed together. Among the curlies, hair shrinkage when the hair is dry is most pronounced with this hair type. Its natural tendency is to frame and hug the head rather than hang downward. Kinky-curly hair, the most fragile of all hair types, is strongest when it has not been chemically straightened.

Chemically-Relaxed Hair

Relaxed hair is kinky-curly hair that has been permanently straightened by chemical means. Special care is required to keep relaxed hair in optimal condition. This hair type is fragile along its length, especially where the straight, chemically treated hair meets the curly "roots" (or new growth) as the hair continues to grow.

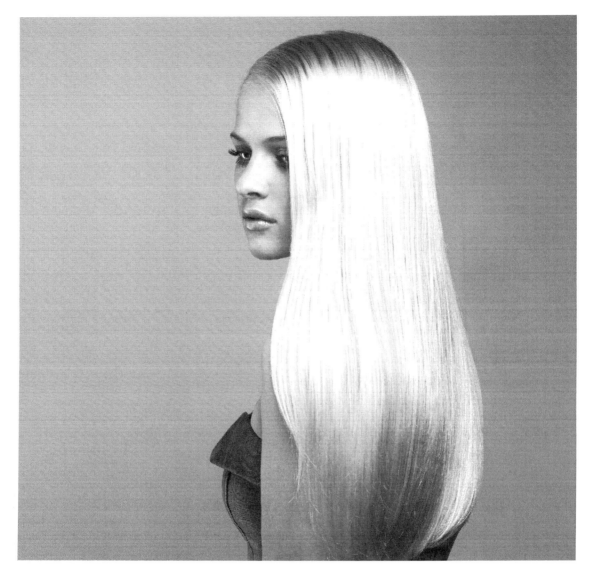

Figure 14- Hair fibers can be classified as straight, wavy, curly and kinky-curly.

Although relaxed hair is breakage-prone, coarser hair fibers tend to stand up to breakage better than fine or medium-textured strands. With a dedicated, healthy hair care regimen in place, this hair type can thrive.

Whether it is chemically straightened or worn in its natural state, kinky-curly hair is almost always matte in appearance and rarely shines—even when it is very healthy.

NOTE: For an in-depth look at the science and care of kinky-curly hair, I recommend picking up a copy of my book, *The Science of Black Hair: A Comprehensive Guide to Textured Hair Care*. The concepts presented in *The Science of Black Hair* go beyond the scope of this guide and are much more technical and targeted than the basic information we can squeeze in here. Check it out!

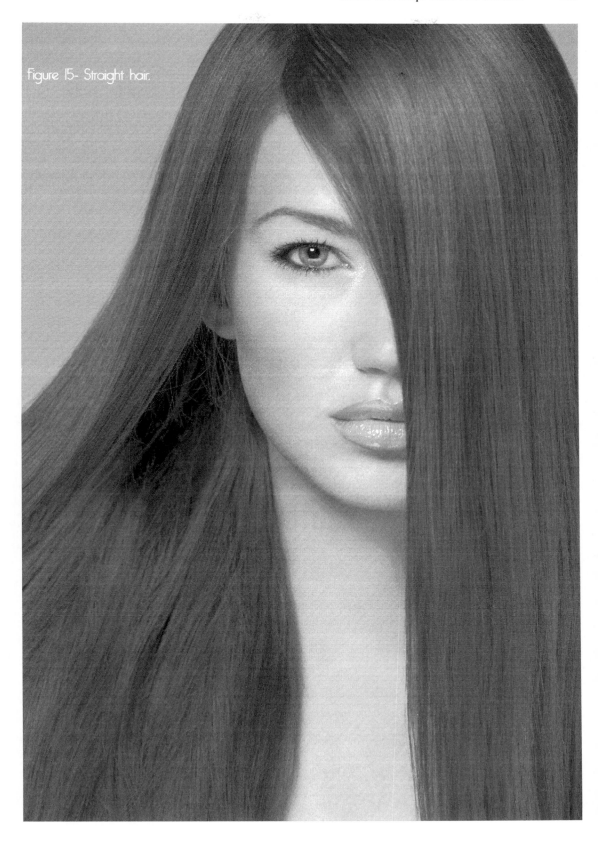

Figure 15- Straight hair.

Figure 16- Wavy hair.

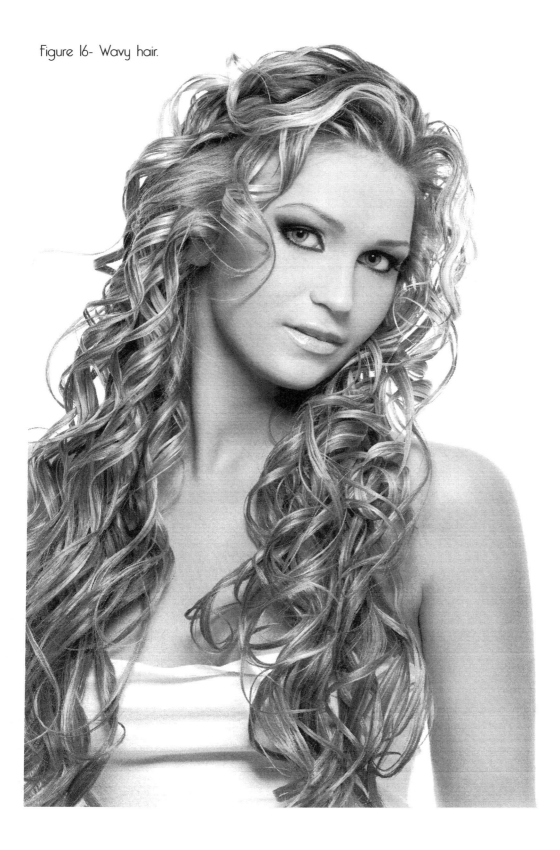

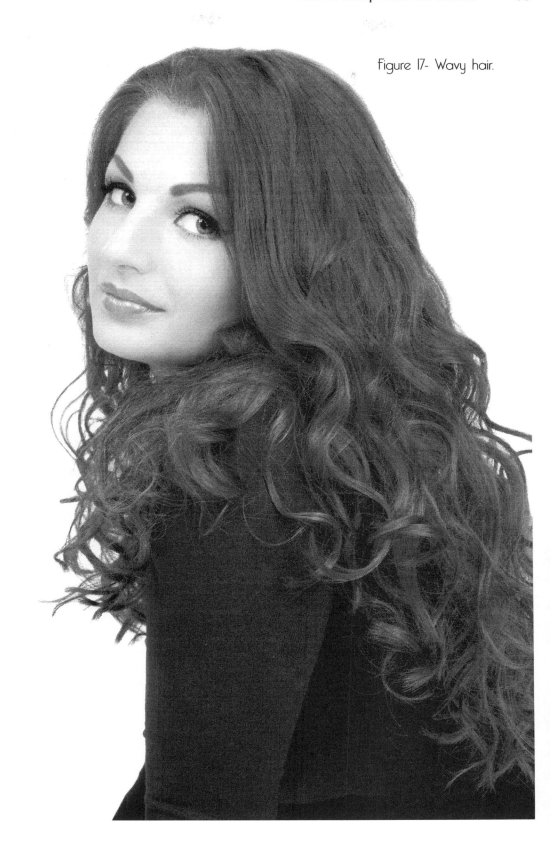

Figure 17- Wavy hair.

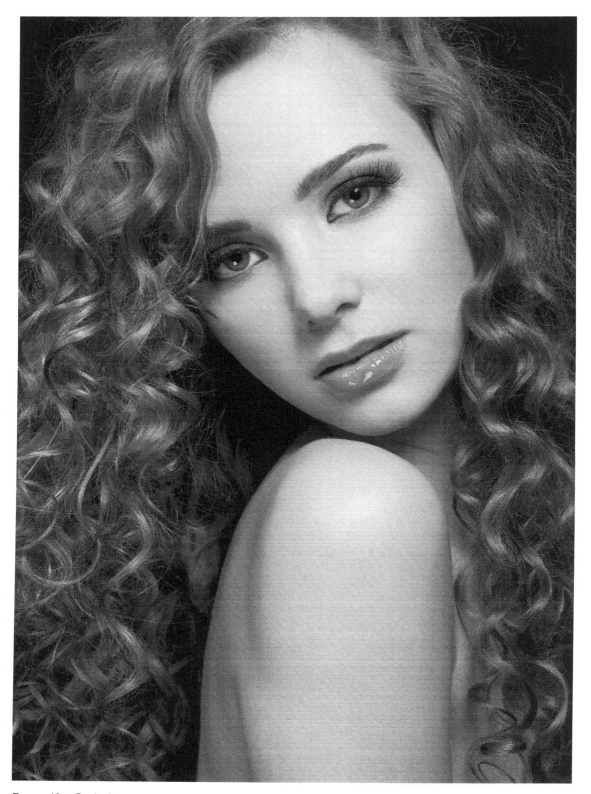

Figure 18- Curly hair.

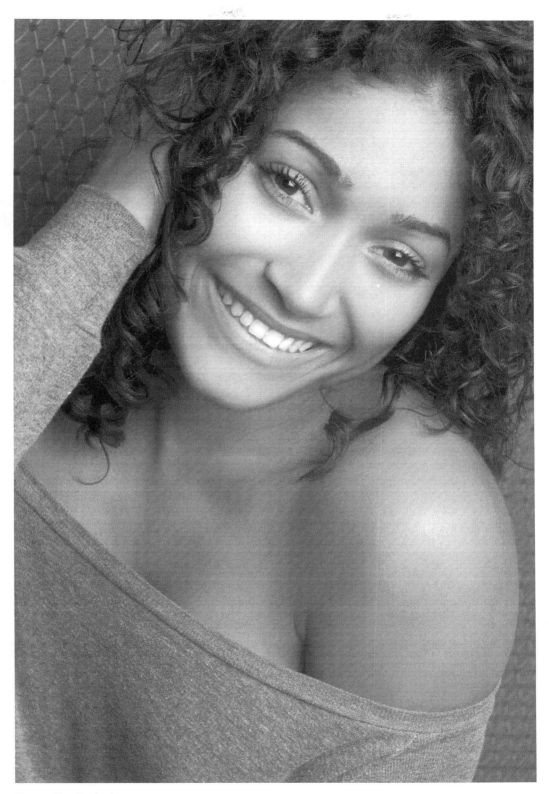

Figure 19- Curly hair.

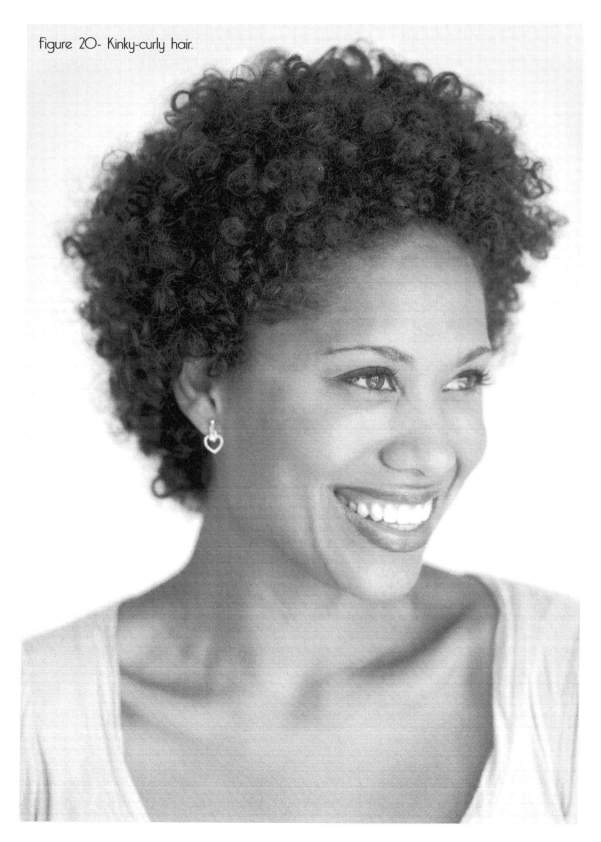

Figure 20- Kinky-curly hair.

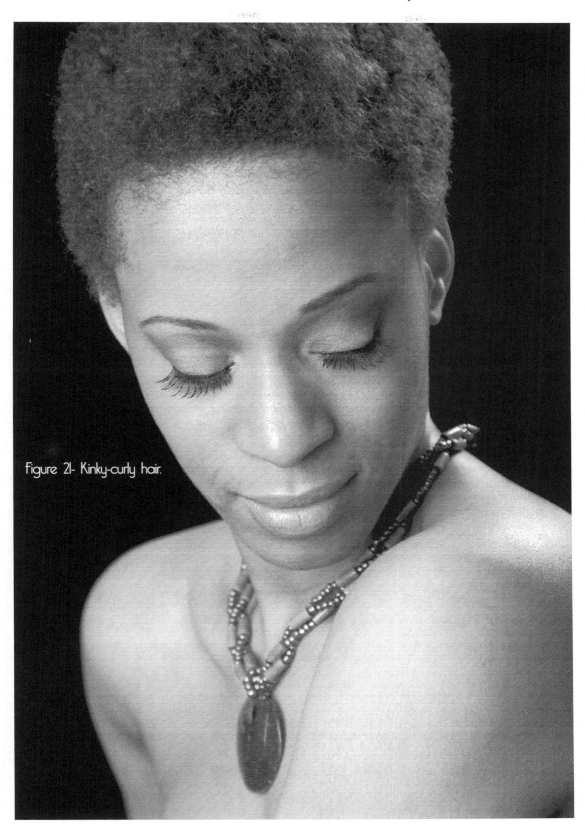

Figure 21- Kinky-curly hair.

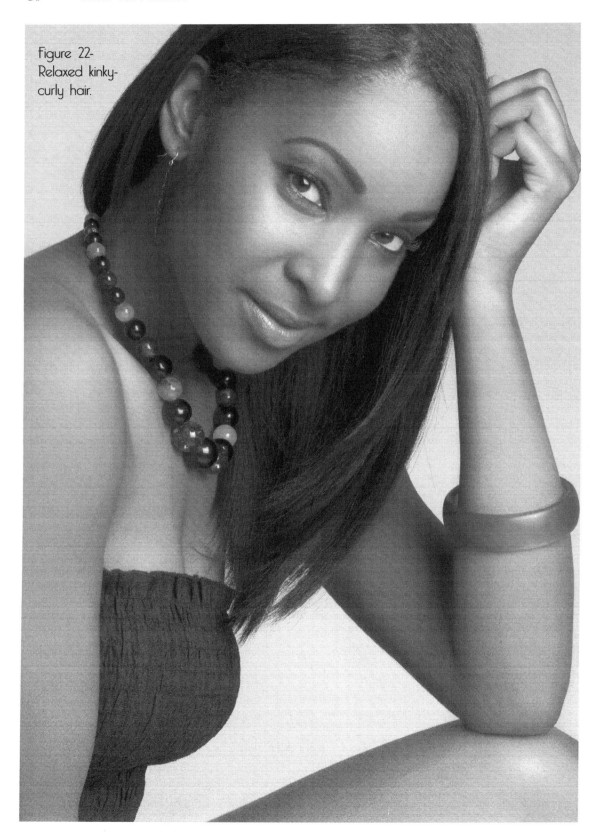

Figure 22-
Relaxed kinky-
curly hair.

Scalp: Just the Basics!

For many people, the scalp is the source of most of their hair problems. And when we look at how many things can affect the scalp's functioning and performance, we can easily see why. Our scalp skin is quite sensitive to everything from the hair products and treatments we use to shifts in our health and hormone levels. Our scalp is even responsive to the changes in weather and environment around us.

Hair products and topical hair treatments can create thick, obtrusive layers on the scalp skin that prevent it from functioning properly. Dehydrated, undernourished bodies produce dehydrated and poorly nourished scalp skin, and changes in the environment from the hot summer months to the bitter-cold winter months can cause our scalps to respond with tightness, dryness, itchiness, and discomfort.

Exploring the Scalp

The scalp is divided into three layers: the *epidermis* (uppermost), *dermis* (middle), and *subcutaneous* (bottom) layer. The subcutaneous layer houses the scalp's dense supply of blood vessels and fatty tissue. The dermis, or middle layer, contains a network of collagen protein that lends strength and support to the skin. The uppermost layer, or epidermis, is roughly fifty cells thick and is the layer we see and work with on a daily basis. It is the very top of this final layer (the *stratum corneum*) that is most important, since it is the layer most affected by all of the skin-flaking disorders such as seborrhea, dandruff, and dermatitis.

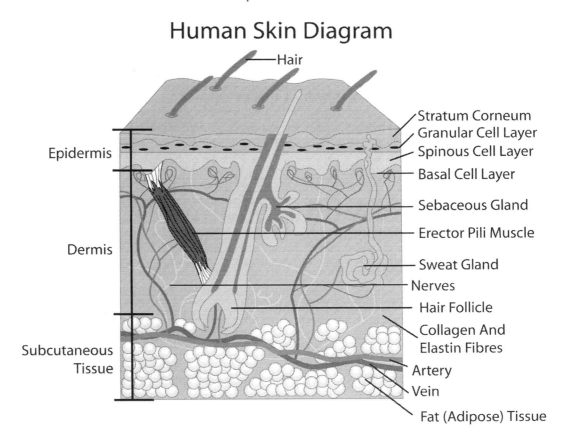

Human Skin Diagram

Figure 23- Diagram of human skin.

Like skin cells all over the body, the cells on the surface of the scalp naturally shed as new cells form. Every day, these scalp skin cells shed as tiny particles invisible to the naked eye.

Water stored in the deeper skin layers slowly migrates toward this uppermost layer of skin to provide moisture and hydration to the skin's surface. Unfortunately, moisture in the uppermost levels of skin soon evaporates into the surrounding environment. This evaporation eventually leaves the scalp skin feeling quite dry. Dandruff and dry, scaly scalp form when the moisture content of the scalp skin drops below 10 percent.

As many of you probably know firsthand, scalp issues in particular can be tricky to manage. They can be difficult to treat because scientists are still trying to pinpoint the exact causes of many of these issues. Today, many skin problems still have no real, effective, long-term cures. Not only do they leave us scratching our heads (literally, right?), they can be expensive to treat over the long term. While total cures are not often possible, establishing some level of relief or comfort for scalp issues often is achievable.

Chapter 2 Rehab Recap

Hair & Scalp: Just the Basics
- Hair is made up of two and sometimes three layers: the cuticle, cortex, and medulla.
- The cuticle layer determines whether or not our hair looks healthy.
- There are three basic hair textures: fine, medium, and thick/coarse.
- Texture is different from hair density. Texture is all about your strand size, while density explains the amount of hair on your head.
- There are four basic hair shapes: straight, wavy, curly, and kinky-curly/coily.
- The scalp is divided into three layers: the epidermis (uppermost), dermis (middle), and subcutaneous (bottom) layer.

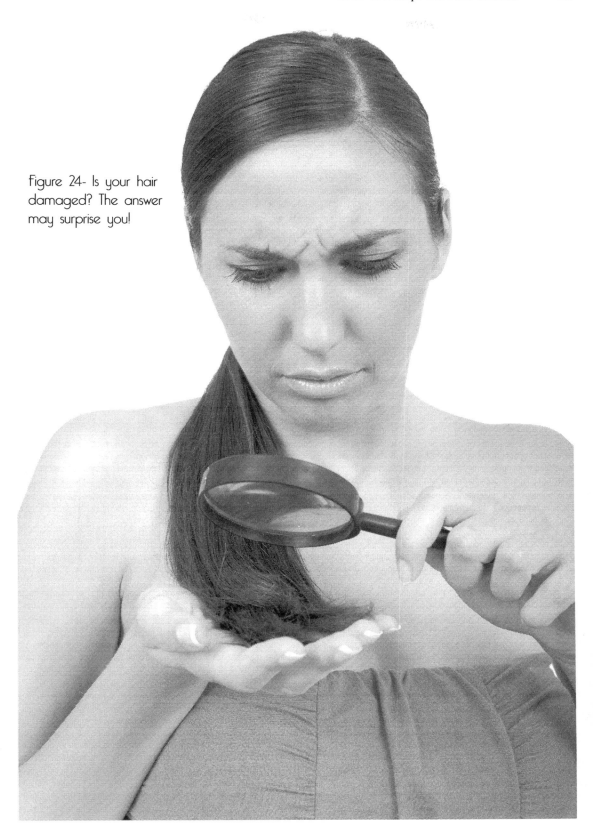

Figure 24- Is your hair damaged? The answer may surprise you!

Chapter 3:
Damage Defined

So, what if I were to tell you that no matter who you are—curly girl, wavy lady, or straight-haired chick—no matter what your hair care practices, no matter how you actually wear or style your hair, *your beautiful hair is irreparably damaged?* You would think I'm crazy—but it's true! *(About your hair, that is!)* Without ever seeing your hair or knowing you or your hair care habits, I can tell you with **100 percent** certainty that your hair is damaged. Long, short, color-treated, natural, or otherwise—your hair is definitely damaged.

And mine is too.

Now, before we get into the juicy stuff, let's first get some important definitions out of the way. What is healthy hair exactly?

What Is Healthy Hair?

Everyone knows what healthy hair looks like. For some, it's simply hair that has great sheen, shine, or length. For others, it's thick, lush, sleek, or bouncy tresses. No matter how you choose to define it, most people will agree that healthy hair has a certain look and quality to it. We know it when we see it! However—despite its outward appearance—our hair does not truly have "health" in the usual sense of that word.

This absence of true health is complicated by the fact that in reality, under the scrutinizing eye of the microscope, all hair is damaged in some way. *All hair.* Damage goes much deeper than what we can readily see. In fact, hair can exhibit none of the traditional signs of damage and still be quite damaged. *How is this possible?*

It's possible because EVERYTHING damages fragile hair fibers: shirts, scarves, combs, fingernails, air, water, heat, products, becoming blonde or a redhead for the eleventh time—

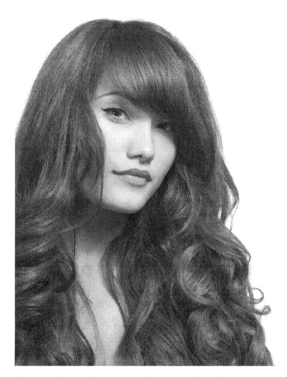

Figure 25- What exactly is healthy hair?

everything. Anything that *touches* the hair has the potential to damage it, never mind the processes (such as coloring and straightening) that are specifically designed to alter its structure! So, when we say our hair is "healthy," we are really just saying that our hair is well-maintained in some aesthetically acceptable state that looks good to the eye and can still accumulate length, despite its imperfect (and technically dead!) condition.

In reality, healthy hair is simply damaged hair that is well-maintained. Now, in the real world, we don't call everyone's hair damaged—for obvious reasons. It is just completely unhelpful to categorize and assess hair damage on a microscale. Case in point: Chemically straightened and color-treated hair is damaged automatically from the start because of the harsh processes that the hair must go through to achieve the final desired result. But someone with lush, shiny, thick

highlighted or chemically straightened hair, or someone with big, voluminous, springy color-treated curls or coils, for example, would not, by most people's standards, have damaged hair. We typically reserve the word *damaged* for hair that is visibly in trouble. This is hair that everyone can see is damaged. It is falling out, shedding erratically, and/or breaking uncontrollably—and it also looks and feels incredibly thin, weak and dry.

Bottom Line?

In *Hair Care Rehab*, we speak of healthy hair from a purely visual standpoint. Because all hair has sustained some level of prior damage, and nonliving fibers cannot truly be said to have "health," we can only really make superficial, cosmetic determinations of perceived health status about our hair from sight and touch. In *Hair Care Rehab*, we define healthy hair as hair that looks, feels, and moves well. The fibers are strong and easily resist breakage with normal manipulation. Simple as that.

What About "Hair Repair"?

Let's talk a little about "hair repair" in general.

Hair repair is the temporary restoration of hair fibers to a "healthy hair" state. Basically, hair that was dull improves in luster or shine, and hair that was limp and brittle regains body and movement. In this book, you should **always understand hair repair to be a temporary hair fix**; the only permanent hair repair solution involves a pair of scissors. Damage to our hair can only be patched up temporarily with conditioners and treatments—and unfortunately, the benefits of patching up our hair generally only last for four to seven days. Why? Because the products we use are usually washed back down the drain with each shampoo-and-conditioning session. Some products with greater affinity for (or chemical attraction to) our hair may be able to withstand a few extra cleansing sessions, but few products and treatments last on the hair beyond a cleansing or two.

Now, hair product manufacturers are really clever. I mean, *really* clever. They will sell you the dream of hair repair as if it's a closed case after you've slathered on their product. Be wary of these sorts of claims. These products simply cover the damage and improve the look of your hair temporarily. The hair repair process is *always* temporary, and treatments must be continued on a regular basis until the damaged hair grows out or is cut off. Although we cannot permanently restore our hair to its original, undamaged condition, the good news is that temporary rebuilding measures *can* significantly improve the look and condition of our hair.

Words, Schmords

Although "healthy hair" and "hair repair" are misnomers, we freely use these terms throughout *Hair Care Rehab* because:

1. They are convenient terms, and

2. Most people understand what they mean.

Instead of repeatedly saying, "Hair that is maintained at some aesthetically acceptable status where it can still accumulate length despite the imperfect condition of the fiber," we will simply say "healthy hair." And rather than speaking about "temporary reconditioning of the fiber to help it maintain this acceptable status," we will say "hair repair." Simple!

The Three Healthy-Hair Requirements

In order for hair to remain healthy and resist hair breakage, the protein and moisture in your hair must be balanced. Our hair strands are made up almost entirely of protein, internally bound moisture, and other binding agents that hold the strand together. (Proteins are chains of amino acids that have been linked together, and moisture is simply water.) In the hair shaft, these protein and moisture components are strongly attracted to one another. (Entire books have been written on this point alone, but I'll spare you and keep it really simple! Just know that the protein and water in our hair must be balanced to keep the hair healthy.)

Our hair's protein and moisture levels control the three hair properties that ultimately determine whether our hair is healthy and breakage-free or hanging on by a thread! A careful mixture of all three of these properties is necessary to have radiant hair.

1. **Elasticity**
Elasticity is the ability of hair strands to bend and flex without breaking. Think of a rubber band. These are highly elastic and can be pulled and stretched a great distance without breaking. When the pulling tension is eased, rubber bands almost always return to their prestretched condition. Healthy hair behaves the same way (but within a shorter range of motion). When hair is stretched out of shape repeatedly, like a rubber band, it will also eventually lose its ability to return to its healthy, prestretched condition. Moisture content is important to ensure a proper level of elasticity.

2. **Porosity**
Porosity is the ability of a hair strand to absorb (and release) moisture, chemicals,

or other products. Hair with high porosity is generally damaged hair. Think of a fence. A fence blocks off a yard to intruders, but some small things are still able to get in and out. Newer fences provide better layers of protection against intrusion, whereas older, worn fences tend to be weaker and allow more things in. Hair that maintains its moisture levels well and accepts color and/or chemical treatments well (if desired) is said to have "good porosity." The protein content of the hair is particularly important here. Protein products help to temporarily fill in damaged areas of the hair shaft (i.e., replace broken planks and boards in the fence).

3. Strength

Strength is a characteristic that is pretty straightforward. The strength of your hair refers to its robustness and its overall resistance to breakage through normal manipulation. Protein content is a major factor here, but moisture also plays a role in the level of trauma a hair may be able to withstand. Parched strands are not strong strands, no matter how much protein reconstruction you do.

If your hair exhibits too much of any of these properties, it will feel weak and eventually break.

Is My Hair Damaged?

So how do you know if your hair is *really* damaged? Test your hair with the following questions:

1. Is your hair breaking?

When our hair is healthy, breakage is minimized almost to the point of nonexistence. There may be occasional periods of breakage, especially when detangling is not handled gently, but for the most part, hair breakage is not a large concern for the healthiest heads of hair.

2. Does your hair have sheen or shine?

The hair's cuticle (the outermost layer of the hair shaft that we discussed in Chapter 2) should lie flat so that light is easily reflected from the hair's surface. The flatter the cuticle's scales, the smoother the surface of the hair strand will be. When the surface is smooth, light can reflect more intensely from the surface, giving us incredible shine. If your hair is curly, coily, or highly textured, your shine will be there—but because of its natural bending and twisting, these types of hair just reflect light in a more scattered, matte kind of way. This type of shine is referred to as "sheen." Shine and sheen should be present from roots to tips. If your hair is damaged, you'll notice less sheen and shine, especially near the ends.

3. Is your hair progressively gaining length?

Unless the hair is intentionally cut, hair should be growing longer over time. Length checks are important, even if growing out your hair is not an immediate goal. Why? Because occasionally, hair breakage occurs so subtly that we are not able to pick up on it as it happens each day. Over time, however, this slow breakage can lead to problems. If we can catch minor problems before they escalate, we can prevent major hair setbacks from occurring. Length checks help us keep our hair healthy overall. *If the length of your hair remains constant over a period of months, there may be unresolved damage from a chronic hair-breakage problem standing in the way of your hair progress.*

Figure 26- Healthy hair must have great elasticity, porosity and strength.

For those with naturally curly or textured hair who prefer not to straighten their hair to check length, you can monitor your progress by simply "pull testing" (pulling a strand to see how long it falls when stretched out completely) or simply monitoring the overall length and volume of your style.

4. Does your hair look full from roots to ends?

Hair may be naturally thick or thin, but relative hair thickness should be somewhat consistent from roots to ends, even with layering. When the hair is straightened, its hemline (the shape that the ends of the hair form naturally along the wearer's back) should remain full. See-through areas, or places of transparency, along the hair's hemline usually indicate areas of damage or unchecked chronic breakage. When hair is damaged, the hair's hemline will have a sharp-edged shape resembling a V or W rather than a rounded, blunt, or U- shape.

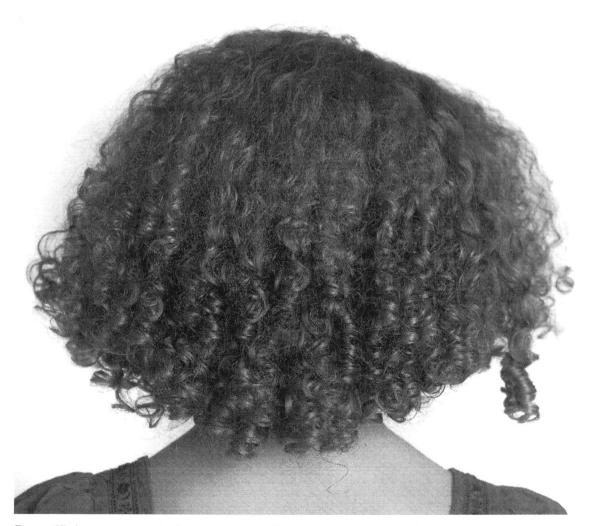

Figure 27- Inconsistent curls from roots to ends can signify damage, but sometimes, it is simply a natural characteristic of the hair.

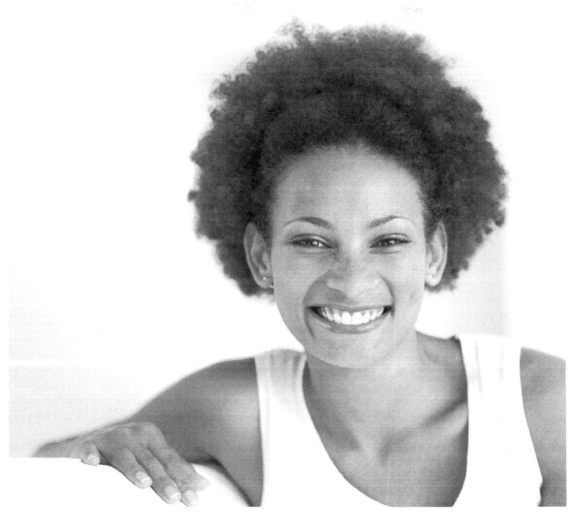

Figure 28- Textured hair can camouflage damage or look damaged when it is quite healthy.

Hair tends to move better when the hair is consistent in its roots-to-ends thickness. There is less friction between individual hair fibers because the cuticle scales are in their healthy tight and flattened position.

5. **Does your hair have consistent color from roots to ends?**

The consistency of the hair's color from roots to ends is also a strong indicator of the hair's condition. Reddened or lightened hair (by this I mean hair that naturally grows in dark but lightens along the length) is a possible sign of damaged hair. This type of lightening that is unrelated to color treatment is also often accompanied by extreme dryness and frizzy or swollen/ puffy hair shafts.

Damage to Curly, Coily & Textured Hair Types

If you're a naturally curly or coily girl, pinpointing hair damage can be a bit trickier. Unlike straight hair, which lends itself easily to visual health inspection, our eyes cannot be as easily trusted to pinpoint damage in hair worn in its curly state.

Some curly hair types look very dry, even though they are completely moisturized and conditioned, and this is particularly true for those with the tightest, coiliest hair types.

The issue is complicated by the fact that although naturally curly hair can look damaged when it is quite healthy, it can also appear healthy when it is in trouble. Curly hair does not show the damage it has sustained as readily as straight hair because the damage is often masked by the hair's texture, volume, and organic shape. There are no reliable areas of transparency along curly hair's hemline (unless the hair is straightened) to reveal a damaged state.

Healthy curly/coily hair should

1. Have minimal breakage. Breakage at any time is an indication of damaged or weakened hair fibers.

2. Have sheen or shine, especially when held taut. Most curly and coily girls will have sheeny rather than shiny curls.

3. Feel strong yet soft, fluffy, and/or springy. Hair that feels dry, scratchy, rough, or hard is very likely damaged.

4. Be progressively gaining length or volume.

5. Have curls, spirals, and coils that maintain their curliness from root to tip. Hair that starts curly and then straightens or goes flat in sections, especially near the ends, is likely damaged. However, curls that start flatter from the roots and build curl towards the ends may be perfectly healthy because the weight of the hair may initially distort the incoming curl pattern.

6. Have root-to-ends color consistency. The roots-to-ends color test described above for straight hair is also effective in revealing areas of damage to curly/coily

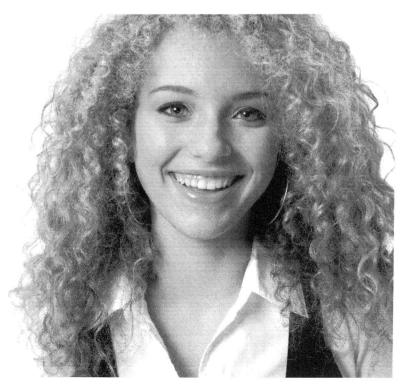

Figure 29- Healthy textured hair should progressively gain length over time.

hair. Any naturally dark hair that lightens toward the ends has been stressed by normal, day-to-day wear and tear.

Hair damage is really just damage to the hair's protein structure that prevents it from being able to reliably keep water or moisture stored securely within the hair fiber. Damaged hair always benefits the most from conditioning because damage to the hair cuticle changes the *outer electrical charge* of the hair fiber. Damaged hair is negatively charged hair—and that's pretty easy to remember if you think, *damage = negative*. Conditioners are positively-charged products that are attracted to hair with a strong negative charge. If your hair is damaged, your conditioner is more likely to have the desired effect on it than if your hair is already healthy.

Chapter 3 Rehab Recap

Damage Defined
- Hair cannot be permanently repaired, only temporarily *reconditioned*.
- Healthy hair is simply hair that has been reconditioned and looks and feels great.
- Healthy hair has good elasticity, good porosity, and good strength.
- Your hair is damaged if it is breaking, lacks shine, doesn't gain length or volume over time, and isn't color-consistent through to the ends.

Chapter 4:

What's Your Drug of Choice?

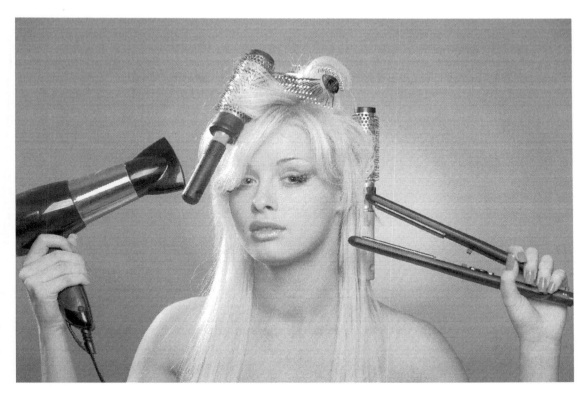

Figure 30- Curling irons, blow dryers, perms—what's your drug of choice?

No matter how well we take care of our hair, we are bound to come face to face with one type of damage or another. Many, many things can affect the health of our hair including age, health status, day-to-day hairstyling techniques, and the environment. If your hair is damaged, it is important to understand how you got there. *What was the final straw? What was your drug of choice?*

Your drug of choice can be nearly any hair practice that has been repeated enough times to stress out, fry, or otherwise destroy your hair into submission. *Was it heat? Too many trips around the color wheel? Careless or forceful hair detangling? General lack of care?* Let's be real here: Coming up with the culprit (or combination of culprits) for your current hair troubles won't be rocket science for you. You know what you've been up to!

The Four Hair Care Drugs of Choice

Now let's take a look at the four basic hair care "drugs of choice" that land many of us in Hair Care Rehab: chemical, physical, environmental, and nutritional abuse. Nearly all hair damage is caused by some combination of these factors!

Chemical Abuse

So platinum blonde was your goal, even though you are a deep-raven or coffee-colored brunette. Your stylist warned you (and you knew better), but you decided to make a go at it anyway. You said to yourself what we all say to comfort ourselves right before we make some crazy hair mistake: *It's just hair . . . it'll grow back.* And you succeeded. You achieved your new color against all odds. Unfortunately, with it came a hefty price-tag for your tresses: an unforgiving, Texas tumbleweed–like dryness!

Chemical processing can cause some of the most devastating types of hair damage, even when products are expertly applied. Of all the hair care addictions, regular chemical services are by far the hardest to kick. The highs can be absolutely beautiful, but the lows—well, you've seen them!

How to Spot an Addict: Addicts will have dull, tangly hair that lacks shine. Their hair tends to feel brittle, unnaturally puffy, or dry—especially near the ends. Hair may also be unnaturally colored, and hair texture and shape may be uneven from root to tip. Abusers may suffer from a form of withdrawal known as "roots" which keeps them trapped in their cycle of dependence.

How Chemical Abuse Happens

1. **Curly Perms**

   - Perm solution left on the hair too long.
   - Incorrect roller size used (usually too small) for hair length and type.
   - Excessive tension placed on rollers during processing (again, usually due to rollers being too small).

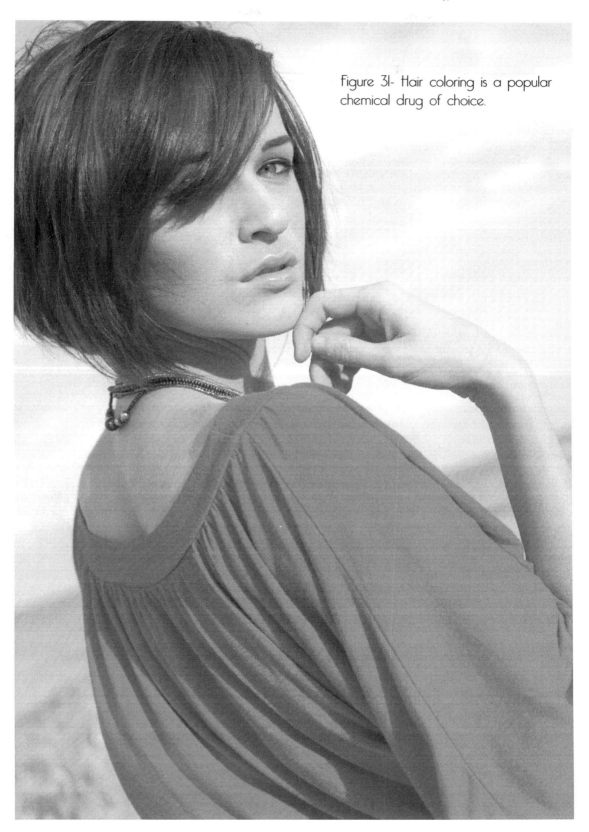

Figure 31- Hair coloring is a popular chemical drug of choice.

- Improper rinsing of perm solution.
- Perming on top of another chemical process.
- Poor aftercare and upkeep.

2. Permanent Color

- New color is more than three shades out of the hair's natural range.
- Hair has been colored many, many times.
- Poor aftercare and upkeep.

3. Chemical Relaxers/Straighteners

- Relaxer strength not appropriate (usually too strong) for hair type.
- Relaxer left on the hair too long.
- Incomplete rinsing with neutralizer solution.
- Poor aftercare and upkeep.

Once chemicals such as curly perms, permanent colors, hydroxide-based relaxers, and texturizers are applied to the hair, the internal structure of the hair shaft is changed forever and cannot be returned to its original state. When these changes happen, our hair's ability to hold important moisture in the fiber also deteriorates. While we often use these styling methods to improve the appearance of our hair, many times they have the opposite effect.

Signs of Abuse

1. Curl pattern & texture changes. While this is desirable for those who are using products such as straighteners or curly perms, when you are color-treating your hair, for example, changing your hair's curl pattern and texture may be the last thing on your mind! Coloring the hair, though, can result in temporary, unpredictable changes

in your hair's curl pattern and texture—and sometimes these changes are permanent. Whenever you alter or manipulate the hair's protein-bonding arrangement, hair swelling and a slight curl-relaxing effect can occur. These changes are more likely to occur in those with fine or medium hair textures. Prior damage may also influence whether or not you experience changes in your curl pattern or texture.

2. Increases in hair porosity. Products that lighten or change the shape of the hair always require direct access to the hair's cortical (innermost) layers. When the hair's cuticle is breached chemically to allow access to the cortex, the hair's natural porosity increases, leading to a dryness that hardly ever lets up. When porosity increases, dryness becomes a major complaint because moisture is next to impossible to hold securely within the fiber. Your hair becomes like a bucket with holes poked in the sides. Chemically-treated hair can be unforgiving, too. Miss a regularly scheduled deep conditioning, and you may find yourself parting with strands prematurely. If you never cared before, now is definitely the time to learn how to balance protein and moisture sources in your regimen!

3. Loss of elasticity. Because chemically treated hair has lost much of its natural moisture (and its overall ability to retain any supplemental moisture it receives), the hair may lose some of its elasticity. Remember: Elasticity refers to the hair's ability to stretch gently and return back to its normal shape and character without damage. The elastic quality of our hair is what makes putting our hair in a ponytail effortless. When hair lacks elasticity, it does not move, bend, and recover when

pressured as healthy hair does; in its fragile condition, it simply gives up under pressure and snaps. Again, moisture and protein balancing becomes critical for reestablishing elasticity because it's that careful mix of moisture and strength that gives our hair the ability to resist breakage.

4. **Unpredictable results.** Chemicals are very, very unpredictable, and all the swatches, box comparisons, and focus groups in the world can't prepare you for the end result that you can expect. Why? Because chemical uptake and turnout depend upon a number of factors, namely your hair's current condition, porosity, and texture (strand size). The color or final result depicted on the hair color box, for example, is just the product manufacturer's best corporate guess at what your hair will look like after using their product—with a bit of "Photoshopping" thrown in for good measure. Sometimes, multiple corrective steps will be needed to get your desired results.

The amount of chemical damage your hair experiences from processing greatly depends on the knowledge and experience of the individual performing the chemical process, your aftercare skills, the characteristics of the product, and how often you process your hair.

Remember: All permanent chemical alterations, no matter how well executed, render some degree of internal damage to the hair fiber, and most chemical processes also irritate the scalp. To top it off, chemical alterations almost always place users in a dependent situation where the process needs to be repeated on a certain schedule to avoid the very obvious (re)appearance of untreated "roots" (new growth)—or even additional breakage in some cases. (*How many of us are willing to tolerate chemical withdrawal in the form of those telltale roots?*) Using these services in the correct frequency for your own personal situation (often less often than manufacturers tend to suggest or even not at all) is always advisable and will help you avoid further damaging your chemically-treated hair.

Obviously, the best way to reduce chemical damage is to limit your exposure to chemicals. This may mean applying hair colors less often or working with colors within your natural color range. If your hair is chemically straightened, it could mean gradually stretching out the frequency of your straightener applications from six weeks to ten or more weeks.

Tips for Functioning Addicts

- Know the risks! Chemically-treated hair is very sensitive to things that you may have taken for granted before (i.e., water, the sun, heat, etc.). Be prepared for added responsibility.
- Never chemically treat your hair on a whim or without a game plan for aftercare.
- Work with an experienced stylist for major chemical services. If you want to go it alone, decide if you *really* trust yourself enough to make these changes on your own. Be honest! *Do you really know what you are doing? What if the process is unsuccessful? Are you prepared for breakage or a less than stellar turnout?*
- Don't let your chemical service appointment be the first time that you sit in your chosen stylist's chair— especially if the change you are contemplating is a drastic one. You want someone who knows you and your hair and who'll be available if you have questions.
- Be real with yourself. If you are lazy, put down the box, *do not pass Go, and do not collect $200!* Chemically-treated hair REQUIRES upkeep, or you will quickly find it circling its way down the drain.

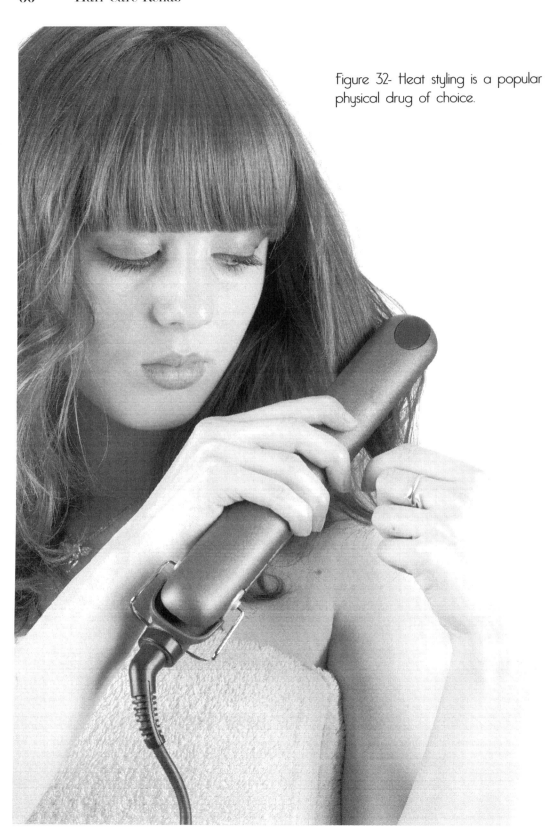

Figure 32- Heat styling is a popular physical drug of choice.

Physical Abuse

There's no denying that ultrastraight hair is your thing. You fire up your irons every morning to achieve that sleek, pin-straight look, and God help the slightest bit of humidity that dares enter the air around you! You're a pro at it, too. Curls and frizz don't stand a chance when you're working your flatiron magic! That is, until one day, when a quick inspection of your ends reveals the honest truth: Your ends are split and fried to high heaven!

How to Spot an Addict: Addicts will have dry, breaking hair that is full of split ends. Although the hair is usually short (not by choice) and probably thin and/or missing in places, some addicts with durable hair types may still manage to grow their hair quite long.

How Physical Abuse Happens

1. Heat straightening and styling.

2. Daily overhandling. Too much combing and brushing, and then recombing and brushing. *A hundred strokes a day, anyone?*

3. Regular, careless towel drying with rough, brisk movements.

4. Wearing ponytails, extensions, and braided or twisted styles that are too tight.

5. Using combs with very small teeth and/or unforgiving seams along the teeth.

6. Using rubber bands and/or ponytail holders with metal pieces.

7. Wet brushing.

8. Sliding rough hairpins, clips, and clamps through the hair repeatedly—in the same locations.

Physical hair damage is caused by incorrect or excessive manipulation of the hair. It is often compounded by stress from other types of hair damage as well.

In the physical abuse category, heat straightening is by far the most commonly used hair care drug of choice. While some resilient hair types are able to withstand daily flatironing, blow drying, or curling, most hair types falter over time. If you are reading a book called *Hair Care Rehab*, chances are, *you* are not in this "strands of steel" category! Most of us can't keep up with such a rigorous styling schedule and high-maintenance routine without falling victim to splits, dryness, and flyaways. (More on heat damage in the Hair Repair Manual, page 186).

Signs of Abuse

1. **Curl pattern, texture & color changes.** Chemical drugs of choice, as we have discussed, usually cause curl pattern, texture, and color changes as *intended* results, but physical hair damage can *unintentionally* lead to these problems. Processes such as heat straightening, very much like chemicals, affect the hair's protein-bonding arrangement and can lead to undesired lightening and loss of natural wave or curl pattern. These changes are more likely to occur in those with fine to medium hair textures because there are fewer layers of cuticle shielding to protect the hair.

2. **Increases in hair porosity.** Physical drugs of choice including heat styling, overcombing and overbrushing can also increase the hair's porosity by scorching, scratching, nicking, bending, and roughing up the hair's cuticle. When porosity increases, dryness becomes a problem.

3. **Breakage & splits.** When physical manipulation goes on unchecked, breakage

to the hair fiber is common. Hair can only handle so much washing, drying, pulling, stretching, wrapping, and winding before it gives up!

Tips for Functioning Addicts

- Know the risks! Save high-manipulation styling choices for special occasions.
- Before brushing or combing the hair, soften it first by applying a small amount of conditioning product (water/moisturizer or oil). This reduces friction between your hair and the styling tool and between individual hairs.
- Limit combing and brushing to no more than once or twice daily. Work with your fingers whenever possible to smooth and arrange hair that is tousled or out of place. If your hair is curly or kinky-curly, you can go a few days between actual combings. Brushing curls should be avoided almost entirely. Finger fluffing or finger combing is the preferred method for working with curls.
- Eliminate wet brushing—or keep it down to a bare minimum using a soft-bristled brush.
- Use a seamless, large-toothed shower comb or wavy-toothed detangler comb to reduce combing damage. These combs are gentle detanglers that work well for all hair types.
- Dry hair with a microfiber towel, carefully squeezing and releasing the hair in a milking fashion, to absorb excess water.
- Air dry or reduce heat use as much as possible. On already conditioned hair, use a diffuser (the attachment that spreads air rather than concentrates it) or hooded dryer to dry the hair. Always use proper heat protection before firing up your appliances. You can find a few great heat protectant products listed in Chapter 8.

Environmental Abuse

Long days outdoors, fun in the sun—and you are totally living summer to the fullest! You love the gentle highlights of sun-kissed hair, taking cool dips in the pool, and nothing can compare to the softness and body your hair has after you've spent a gorgeous, salty day on the sea. Unfortunately, these relatively innocent outdoor plans can also mean dry, straw-like, and even green hair for some of us!

How to Spot an Addict: Addicts will have dull, tangly hair that lacks shine and tends to feel brittle. Hair may be unnaturally reddish if it is naturally darker in color (or a brassier blonde, if the hair is naturally lighter). Color changes are most noticeable near the ends of the hair.

How Environmental Abuse Happens

1. Regular sun exposure.

2. Swimming in heavily chlorinated swimming-pool water or salty ocean water without proper hair precautions and protection.

3. Washing hair in hard water (water with high concentrations of dissolved minerals).

4. Extreme weather and climate scenarios (too arid or too cold).

5. Pollutants and irritants present in the atmosphere, water, and our products.

Whether it's your tap water or harsh UV rays breaking down your hair's proteins, these environmental drugs of choice can leave the hair feeling weaker and damaged.

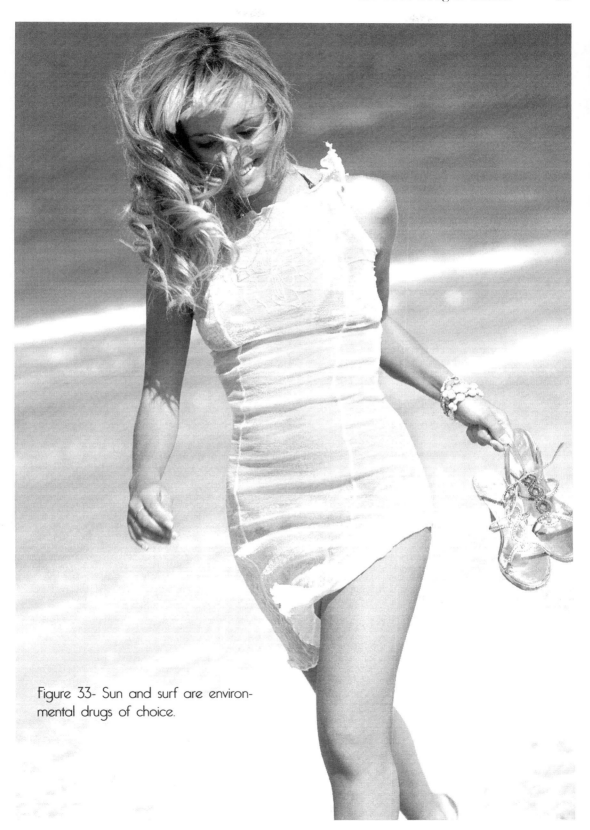

Figure 33- Sun and surf are environmental drugs of choice.

Signs of Abuse

1. **Curl pattern, texture & color changes.**
    As with chemical drugs of choice, which
    most often produce curl pattern, texture,
    and color changes as *intended* results,
    environmental hair damage can also
    change the look and feel of our hair and
    can even fade our natural hair color. The
    color-change effect is amplified on wet
    hair and on hair that has been previously
    chemically-treated.

2. **Increases in hair porosity.** Since sun
    exposure can break down the hair's
    cuticle protection, it always increases our
    hair's natural porosity. This effect is also
    amplified on wet hair and on hair that has
    previously been chemically-treated. When
    porosity increases, we are always left with
    dryness. Dryness is also compounded in
    hard-water situations because of mineral
    "scale" (deposits) left on the outside of the
    hair fiber.

Tips for Functioning Addicts

*   Know the risks! Cover and protect your
    hair from the sun when you'll be outdoors.
    Give your hair a touch of sunscreen before
    heading outdoors if you'll be outside for a
    while.
*   Have your water tested for hardness. You may
    need to pick up a water filter to help soften
    your water.
*   Wear a swim cap or coat your hair with
    conditioner prior to getting into a swimming
    pool or other body of water.
*   Braid your hair or secure it in a ponytail to
    prevent tangles when you're out of the water.
    Loose hair can be "Tangle City" when you're
    exiting a pool!

You'll get great tips in the Hair Repair Manual
section of this book (Chapter 6) for dealing with
this hair care drug of choice!

Nutritional/Dietary Abuse

Unless you are one of the few people who really
monitor what goes in and out of their bodies,
you can count poor diet as a very popular drug
of choice. We're the microwave generation alright.
We want our food sooner rather than later, and
honestly, how many of us can say that we truly eat
well-balanced meals at every single sitting? When
was the last time you ate a vegetable that wasn't in a
box or can? And when we aren't stuffing ourselves,
we're dieting, which can sometimes lead to a lack
of vital nutrients in our diets. Keeping your diet
balanced between the major food groups ensures
the proper functioning of your hair follicles.

Thyroid disorders, anemia, smoking, crash or
restrictive-food-group dieting, and a host of other
factors reduce the overall quality of the hair we
produce. While the best nutrition comes from
the foods we eat, a daily multivitamin is great
for supplementing your diet if your food intake
is less than ideal.

How to Spot an Addict: Addicts will have dry,
weak, or limp hair that is probably thinning.
There may be some actual hair loss, and hair
growth is generally very sluggish.

How Dietary Abuse Happens

1. Fad or crash dieting.

2. Restrictive-food-group dieting.

3. Low water consumption.

4. Smoking.

5. Untreated health conditions including
    anemia or thyroid disorders.

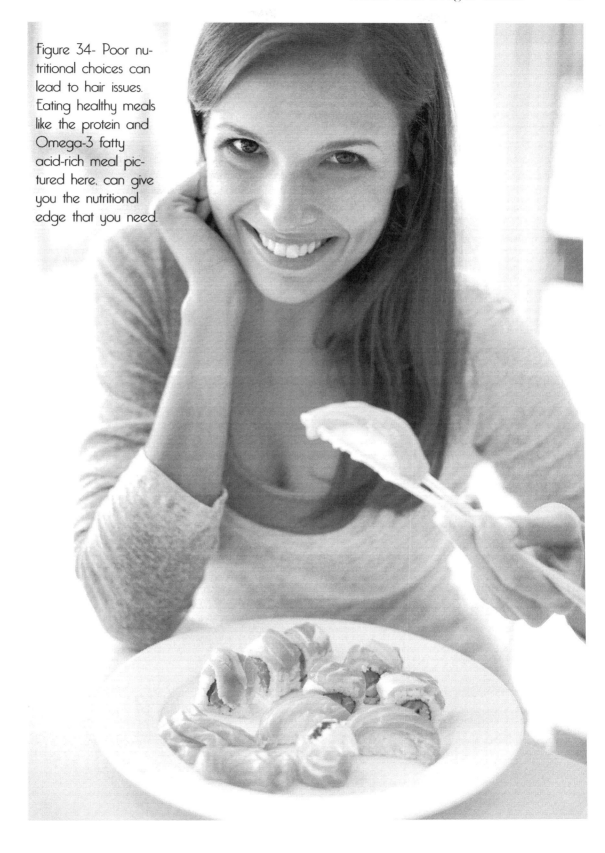

Figure 34- Poor nutritional choices can lead to hair issues. Eating healthy meals like the protein and Omega-3 fatty acid-rich meal pictured here, can give you the nutritional edge that you need.

Our hair can tell us quite a bit about our overall health. *Have you ever seen a sickly, undernourished person with amazing hair? Probably not!* The cells that make up our hair are among the fastest growing in the body, so when the body is in trouble, hair is one of the first places to show it (skin, too).

Your body is organized and has priorities. Unfortunately, hair is pretty low on the list. For your body—the decision between keeping the heart pumping properly, and providing the hair with ultimate strength and gloss, is pretty much a no-brainer! Your body will invest energy into mission-critical areas first.

So without question, we should strive to have a healthy body first—so that the healthy hair and scalp will fall into place. Dietary and nutritional deficiencies can negatively impact the hair before it ever emerges from the scalp, so maintaining the right balance of vitamins and minerals is crucial. Once nutritional deficiencies are corrected, the hair will begin to thrive again.

Signs of Abuse

1. **Curl pattern, texture & color changes.** Nutritional deficiencies can also lead to gradual changes in the hair's curl pattern, color, and texture. Weak, brittle hair shafts and graying or inconsistent color are not uncommon when the body's dietary intake is subpar.

2. **Breakage & hair loss.** When nutritional imbalances are not dealt with effectively, chronic breakage can become a problem. Some hair loss at the scalp level may also occur when hair follicles are undernourished or are affected by medication.

NOTE: The intake of some acne medications, diet pills (with amphetamines), and some cancer

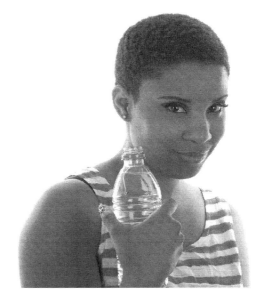

Figure 35- Increasing water intake can improve the quality of the hair you produce.

therapies may also lead to hair damage and loss. If you are taking a medication that may be adversely affecting your hair, do not end your treatment unless advised by your doctor. He or she may be able to provide alternative treatment plans for your condition if you share your concerns.

Tips for Functioning Addicts

- Know the risks! Work with your medical provider to find a diet plan that works for you and your situation.
- Ensure you get adequate protein! Hair is protein, so your diet should include proteins which can be found naturally in meat, fish, poultry, eggs, milk products, tofu, many vegetables, beans, rice and seeds.
- Keep your diet supplied with a good balance of L-lysine (found in chicken, beef, lentils and beans), iron (found in dark leafy veggies, fish and red meat), and vitamins A (found in meats, carrots, milk, cheese, eggs, dark leafy veggies, apricots, papayas, watermelons and mangos), B-complex (found in eggs, rice, milk, and

grains), and C (found in citrus fruits, broccoli, cauliflower, bell peppers and tomatoes). Eating a "rainbow palette" of fruits and vegetables will help you cover most of your dietary needs.
- Consider taking a multivitamin to supplement vitamins and minerals that cannot be obtained from food. The catch to this is that vitamins and minerals are best absorbed when the body is already healthy and the diet is balanced.
- Reduce caffeine and processed sugar intake.
- Stop smoking, and be sure that you are receiving treatment for any underlying medical issues you have.

Chapter 4 Rehab Recap

What's Your Drug of Choice?
- Hair damage occurs whenever we indulge in certain hair care drugs of choice.
- The top drugs of choice are:

 1. Chemical (perms, relaxers, colors).
 2. Physical (combing, brushing, heat use).
 3. Environmental (sun, surf, air, water).
 4. Nutritional/dietary (fad diets, smoking, low water consumption).

- One or a combination of these four drugs of choice can land you in Hair Care Rehab!
- Eliminating or phasing out those damaging factors will get you back on the road to success.

Once you pinpoint your drug (or drugs) of choice, simply eliminate or phase out those damaging factors from your hair care regimen. Which drug of choice has resulted in the current poor state of your hair?

Unit II:
The Detox

n. dee-toks

treatment designed to rid the hair, mind, and body of
harmful substances and practices.

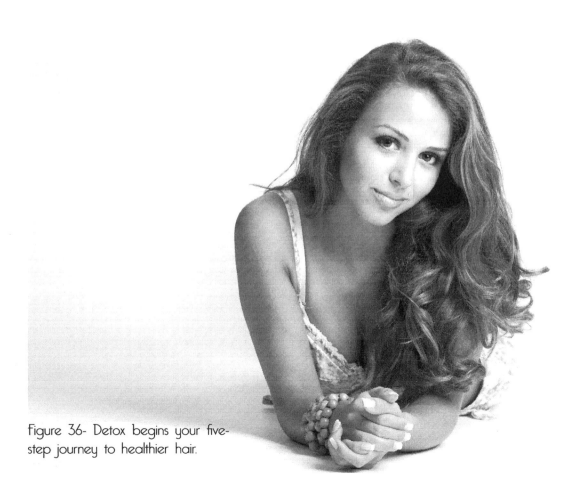

figure 36- Detox begins your five-
step journey to healthier hair.

Chapter 5:
Getting Damage under Control

We know what makes hair healthy and happy. *Check.* We understand how to assess damage. *Check.* And we've just read up on basic hair structure and key properties to guide us through rehab. *Check.* But you may be asking yourself, *How do I get myself back on track? What do I do if I'm not sure where to start with hair care in general?* You are pretty sure your hair is in bad shape, but hair care may as well be high-energy particle physics to you. You just need something simple to follow to keep your hair on your head. If your hair product selection process is pretty much based upon which shampoo matches your bathroom décor or which conditioner smells the fruitiest, then we're about to revamp your thinking! Hang tight—*Hair Care Rehab* has got you covered. We'll run you through the basic techniques and products you need to keep your hair looking great!

The Five-Step Healthy-Hair Detox Regimen

If your hair is very damaged or is experiencing considerable breakage, it is important for you to go through *hair care detox* before incorporating any new hair care methods or solutions. In Hair Care Rehab, this means you'll need to go for a short time without (or minimize the use of) your hair care drug(s) of choice. Sure, you may suffer a bit of withdrawal, which can last a few days

or a few weeks, but the end result? Incredibly healthy hair!

Detox is a five-step process that will help you establish a healthy hair baseline. For best results, the regimen should take place over four weeks. During detox, we get any damage that we have caused to our hair under control, so that we can begin a new chapter in its care. The ultimate, and perhaps easiest, form of detox is to simply cut the damaged hair.

Figure 37- Learn how to regain control of your hair!

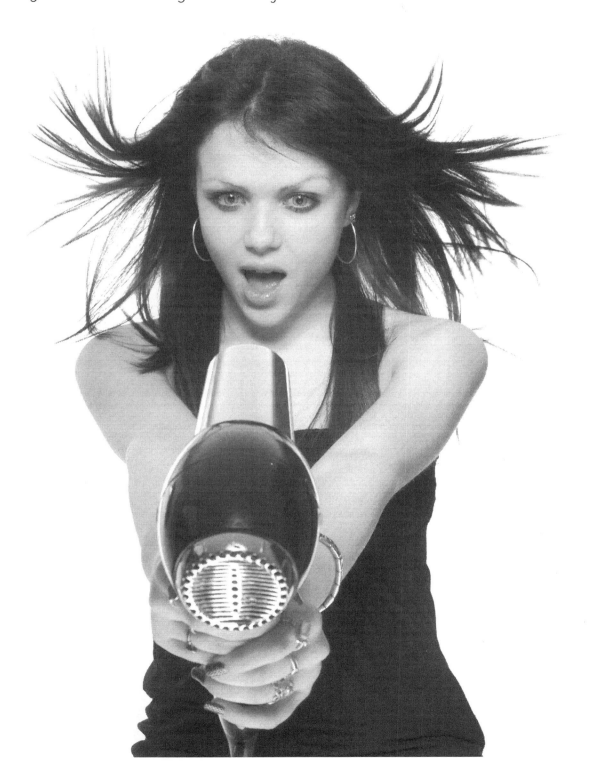

But, if you're not willing to undergo drastic measures, the following Five-Step Healthy Hair Detox Regimen can form the basis of your future hair care routine and jumpstart your hair repair.

Basic Hair Detox Consists of Five Key Steps:

1. Chelating your hair.

2. Deep conditioning your hair.

3. Moisturizing your hair.

4. Sealing your hair.

5. Protectively styling your hair.

This regimen addresses the hair's elasticity, porosity, and strength requirements through a four-week protein- and moisture-balancing conditioning strategy to stop the cycle of damage. Although this regimen works well for nearly every hair type and situation, those with fine, oily or easily weighed-down hair may need to adjust the Healthy Hair Detox Regimen to meet their styling needs.

Hair's recovery from excessive damage can take anywhere from one to four weeks, depending upon the level of damage sustained and how dedicated you are to your repair regimen. Keep in mind that severe damage cases may not respond to temporary cosmetic fixes at all and may require a trim or cut. Just as it takes time for your hair to become damaged, it may take time to see healthy-hair results. If you are patient and dedicated to the process, you'll be okay.

Let's go through each step!

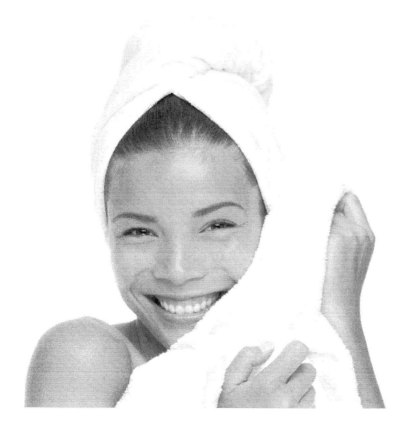

Figure 38- Ready for detox? Let's go!

Step 1: Cleanse Your Hair

Rehab R$_x$

Step I: Cleanse your hair to remove stubborn buildup from products and hard water.

Weeks 1-4

During the first rehab cleansing, use a chelating shampoo* to cleanse and lift stubborn minerals, oils, and debris from the hair. For cleansings after the start-up wash, use a sulfate-free daily shampoo or moisturizing shampoo to clean the hair. You may wash your hair as often as you like each week—but be sure to wash at least once every week.

* If a chelating shampoo is not available, work with a clarifying shampoo instead. For a full list of product recommendations, see On the Shelf!, page 260.

It's certainly true that we humans have a preoccupation with being clean. This probably explains why shampoo is purchased and used by more people than any other hair product on the market! Shampooing plays a critical role in healthy hair detox. The goal of shampooing in detox is to free the hair of all buildup from hair products and hard-to-remove minerals deposited there by our water. When products such as oils, conditioners, serums, and pomades—or minerals including calcium and magnesium from hard water—build up on the hair, they can stand in the way of your ability to truly moisturize or hydrate the hair.

To kick off Detox Step I, we'll use a special shampoo known as a chelating (*key-late-ing*) shampoo. Most people have never heard of chelating shampoo, but it is essential to turning damaged hair around. We'll delve more into the various types of shampoos in a bit.

Shampoo

Today's shampoos offer a wide variety of cleansing levels to suit our hair's needs. Between *moisturizing shampoos, 2-in-1 shampoos, clarifying shampoos, chelating shampoos*—it's easy to get lost in the shuffle! Each shampoo serves its own purpose, and depending on your lifestyle and preferences, you may need one or a combination of these cleanser types over a lifetime. It should be noted that while

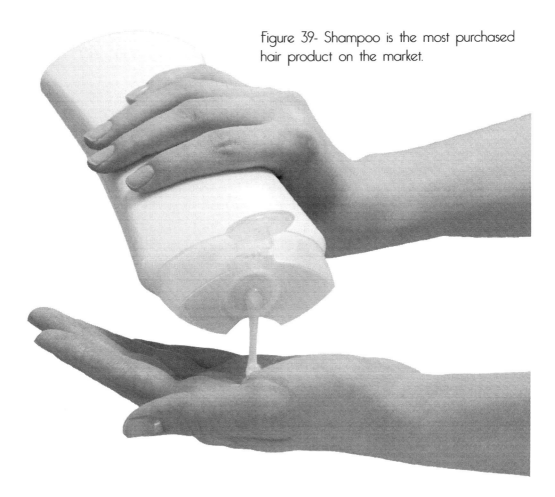

Figure 39- Shampoo is the most purchased hair product on the market.

shampoo remains a staple in most hair care regimens, product formulations are changing so rapidly that even shampoo as a "hair care given" for certain hair types is being challenged. In fact, many curly and/or color-treated girls have abandoned traditional shampoos for simple water rinsing or cleansing with conditioner products. Those who've remained loyal to shampoo are likely using detergent-light, sulfate-free varieties. They are just easier on the hair.

What's in There?
Shampoos contain cleansing agents to lift products, oils, and debris from the scalp. The most common cleansing ingredients in shampoos are the sulfates. Sulfates are harsh detergents that vary in terms of their stripping power. Ammonium lauryl and laureth sulfates (abbreviated as ALS and ALES) are harshest and tend to be the best cleansers, followed by sodium lauryl and laureth sulfates (abbreviated as SLS and SLES) respectively. Sulfate-based ingredients are easy to spot in the ingredients list since they always contain some version of the word *sulfate*. Pretty simple! Check the shampoo bottles in your home; you'll find that nearly all of them contain sulfates. If you've brushed your teeth today, you've probably also used a sulfate-based toothpaste to do that!

Types of Shampoos
Because there are so many different hair types and textures in our world, there is no one shampoo formula that will give everyone healthy hair.

(And, of course, shampoos of different cleansing strengths are often required to achieve various styling goals.) For example, if you've been using firm-hold styling gels, hairsprays, oils, waxes, or glues on your hair, you'll need a high-powered shampoo that can lift these stubborn, weighty products—not a superconditioning formula that will just deposit more oily substances on the hair. If your water is hard or if you are a swimmer, you'll need a special shampoo for that too. Curly or color-treated hair will require more gentle shampoo formulas. How can you quickly tell the difference between a deep cleansing shampoo formula and a rich, moisturizing shampoo formula on the shelf? Well, most of the time, deep cleansing product formulas are *clear*. (They do not contain softening and conditioning ingredients, which typically make a shampoo pearly or opaque). Your lifestyle and hair type will dictate what needs to go under your cabinet.

In Hair Care Rehab, there are four main types of shampoos:

1.) Chelating,

2.) Clarifying,

3.) Moisturizing, and

4.) Daily shampoos.

A fifth type of shampoo (specialty shampoos for dandruff or flaking conditions) also exists, but we'll get to that later on (see Dandruff & Dry Scalp in the Hair Repair Manual, page 139).

Chelating Shampoos

We will kick off rehab by using the most deeply cleansing shampoo formula on the market, the *chelating shampoo*. Chelating shampoos are designed to lift the most stubborn types of buildup from your hair, including the kind that you

can't usually see: mineral buildup from water. Swimmer's shampoos are probably the most widely known type of chelating shampoo, but these deep cleansers can be used for a variety of purposes. This rehab starter cleanse uses them to provide your hair with a clean slate to begin the repair process!

Chelating shampoos are specially formulated to remove mineral deposits that latch onto our hair from hard water and other environmental impurities. Chelating ingredients such as EDTA (ethylenediaminetetra acetic acid), sodium citrate, and trisodium phosphate work to remove those mineral deposits as the hair is rinsed. Since they are such high-powered cleansers, chelating formulas also tend to be sulfate-based. Used too often, these shampoos can be drying to the hair because they easily strip away the natural oils that would normally keep the hair soft and manageable.

While new sulfate-free products are quickly entering the market, most chelating formulas are still sulfate-based. **To avoid issues with dryness during the rehab cleansing step, a moisturizing or volumizing shampoo should take the place of the chelating shampoo after the initial cleansing.**

Clarifying Shampoos

If you do not have access to a chelating formula, a clarifying shampoo formula is your next best bet to kick off rehab! Clarifying shampoos are heavy-duty cleansers that are specially formulated to lift stubborn gels, serums, hair sprays, mousses, pomades, and oils from our hair. Many people confuse clarifying shampoos with chelating shampoos—and it's not that hard to do! The two are similar in that both deeply clean the hair and remove product buildup; but unlike chelating shampoos, clarifying shampoos cannot remove mineral deposits from the hair.

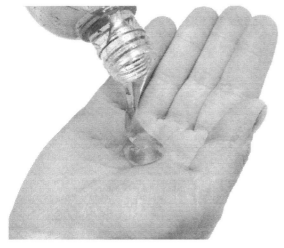

Figure 40- Chelating and clarifying shampoos tend to be clear.

Like most chelating shampoos, clarifying shampoos also leave the hair with a squeaky-clean feeling. These shampoos are great for really oily, fine or lank hair that is easily weighed down. A good clarifier may also be called upon once a month to remove buildup in "product-intense" hair care regimens where lots of oils, hairsprays, polishers and serums are used. These deep-cleansing shampoos will help remove excessively stubborn products and debris that can put up a fight! Used too often, however, these shampoos can be really drying—especially for those with curly, textured and color-treated hair.

Moisturizing Shampoos

Moisturizing shampoos cleanse the hair while leaving behind gentle emollients and conditioners to start the hair-conditioning process. While some may immediately associate moisturizing formulas with limp, weighed down hair, the truth is that we all need shampoo formulas that are gentle and can provide moisture for our hair. The problem with most "moisturizing" formulas on the market, however, is that they "moisturize" by coating the hair in oils and silicones. These rich, creamy formulas are best for medium to thick, curly, color-treated, and severely dry hair

because they help smooth frazzled cuticle layers. But oils, as we will discuss in detail in Step 4, are not actually moisturizers—only water is! So, what do you do if your hair can't handle all of the oily nourishment? What if your hair is fine, but dry or color-treated? Fortunately, getting moisture in your shampoo bottle does not have to mean weighed-down, oily hair; you can still find weightless moisture in a volumizing formula. Many well-formulated volumizing shampoos for fine or oily hair can moisturize the hair without making it flat, limp or greasy.

To sum it up: Thicker, drier hair types need moisture plus heavier coating ingredients to help smooth the hair and retain moisture. Fine to medium and oily hair types need the moisture minus the heavy shaft-coating ingredients so that they maintain volume. The key is to moisturize the hair while still achieving your other styling goals.

Daily Shampoos

Daily shampoos are your standard, run-of-the-mill shampoo. These formulas are generally marketed to those with "normal hair." Shampoos for normal hair are light to medium cleansers. They are best for fine to medium textures because they won't leave oily residues on the hair. Many volumizing shampoos fit into this category. For those with dry, damaged hair, however, these shampoos can be harsh and leave the hair needing more support.

How to Shampoo

We've all seen the shampoo commercials in which models and actresses joyfully fluff soapy balls of hair on the tops of their heads.

Unfortunately, this is a terrible way to clean the hair! It roughs up the cuticle layers and leads to unnecessary tangling—especially for those with long, wavy, curly or highly textured hair. The proper way to cleanse hair is with the strands oriented downward.

If your hair is highly textured or very thick, consider washing your hair in loosely braided sections to keep the hair organized during your wash. This will greatly reduce hair tangling and the amount of hair lost to the cleansing process.

Before shampooing your hair, gently detangle it first using your fingers and a wide-toothed comb if you desire. Gently wet your hair with warm water, and allow the water to free and remove any product buildup from your strands. Carefully squeeze a quarter-size amount of shampoo into your palms and spread it in your hands before lathering it through your hair in a gentle squeezing motion. Rinse well.

Post-Rehab: Choosing a Good Shampoo for Regular Use

Depending on the type of shampoo formula you are using, there may be more or less cleansing power in your bottle. Clarifying and chelating shampoos tend to have more cleansing power (or stripping ability) than moisturizing and daily shampoos. Of course, the more cleansing power your shampoo has, the harsher the formula and the drier it can make your hair feel over time. Shampoos that contain conditioning ingredients to balance their cleansing and conditioning abilities are especially useful for those with dry or textured hair types, but those with fine or oily hair will find their hair weighed down by these formulas. The shampoo you choose (if you use one at all) will always depend on your personal hair type and what you need your shampoo to do.

Shampoos for Thirsty Tresses
Sulfate-free moisturizing shampoos are best for those with coarse, dry, color-treated, or chemically-treated hair and those with curly or

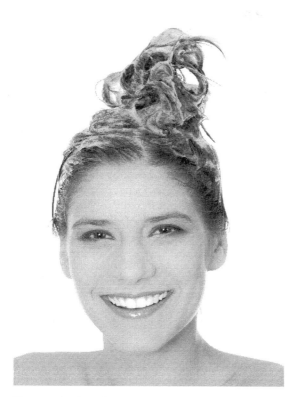

Figure 41- Avoid piling your hair on your head during the cleansing phase.

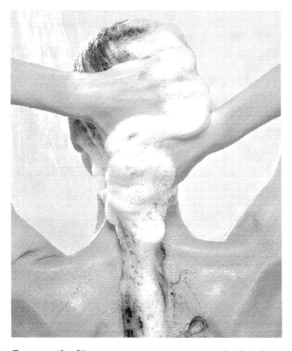

Figure 42- Shampoo your tresses with the hair oriented downward.

highly textured hair. These hair types tend to be dry because the cuticle has been damaged by styling processes or because natural oils simply have trouble making it through the hair. Sulfate-based shampoos can strip moisture and oil that desperately need to be left behind for manageability. Sulfate-based shampoos also fade hair-coloring jobs with lightning speed. With daily or weekly use, these harsh detergents can deplete hair of its vital moisture balance and cause the hair and scalp to feel dry and rough. Moisturizing shampoos are great for use several times each week because they help replenish nourishing emollients along the length of the hair fiber.

Shampoos for Whisper-Fine & Oily Tresses
Naturally fine, oily or straight hair tends to distribute natural scalp oils more efficiently than other types, but can suffer from the opposite problem: greasiness. Most moisturizing shampoos can compound this problem by laying down layers of smoothing agents and oils on the fiber. Shampoo formulas for these hair types should still provide moisture, but without the heavy oils and emollient conditioners. Products should rinse cleanly from the hair so that it does not lose body. Daily shampoos and moisturizing shampoos that volumize and bodify the hair tend to be better options for those needing more regular oil removal.

Step 2: Deep Condition Your Hair

Rehab R$_x$

Step 2: Deep condition your hair.
After the startup cleanse, your hair should be thoroughly deep conditioned with a *moisturizing conditioner** for 10 to 15 minutes. You will only need to deep condition your hair every 7 to 10 days during detox. (If your hair is in serious trouble, every 3 to 5 days may be necessary.) If your weekly shampoo routine includes several cleansings during the week, simply use a basic conditioner formula that rinses cleanly and provides smooth, tangle-free hair for those additional cleansing sessions.

Strive to deep condition with heat, especially if your hair is very damaged. Heat softens the hair and enhances the conditioning and staying power of most conditioner products. Always rinse conditioners with cool water.

NOTE: If your hair is color-treated, using heat to deep condition may fade your color. If your hair is fine and your deep conditioner also volumizes, this may also reduce some of your color's vibrancy.

* In Week 2 or 3, you may need to introduce a protein-based deep conditioner to replace the moisturizing conditioner. Please see pages 83-84 for details on when to make the conditioner switch.

For a full list of product recommendations, see On the Shelf!, page 263.

A great conditioning product is required for success in Detox Step 2. Deep conditioning helps us establish and maintain a baseline level of hair health. As you'll find throughout this book, this simple, often underutilized step is CRUCIAL in healthy hair care. Deep-conditioning treatments are *always* a key factor in turning around hair care problems—in fact, I can't think of one hair condition for which deep conditioning the hair wouldn't be part of the recovery plan. Deep conditioning helps to prevent further damage and enhances the appearance of hair that is

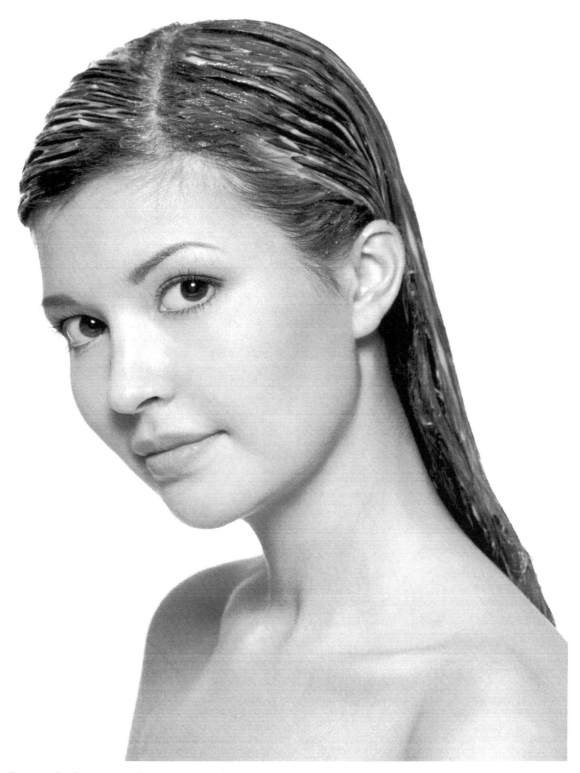

figure 43- Deep conditioning is the heart of any rehab regimen.

already damaged. Hair that is regularly deep conditioned simply responds differently and feels better than hair that isn't kept on a good conditioning schedule. But, not all conditioners are created equal.

Conditioners

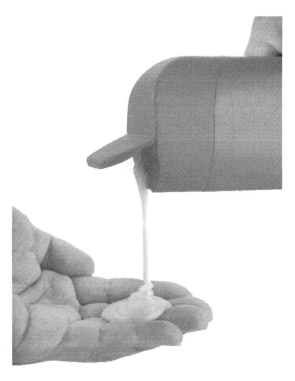

Figure 44- Conditioners provide a layer of protection against hair damage.

The conditioner you select is perhaps the single most important element in your regimen. While the various shampoo products are optional, depending upon your needs, conditioners are rarely up for debate. Conditioners restore moisture lost to the shampooing process and improve the hair's manageability. Because they are meant to adhere to the hair's cuticle and produce effects that remain long after rinsing, conditioners play the most critical role in maintaining the hair's protein/moisture balance. Despite the fact that damage to the hair fiber is always cumulative and

can never be permanently repaired, hair can be conditioned such that split ends are temporarily bonded, cracks are filled in along the cuticle, and a layer of protection exists against further assaults.

What's in There?

Conditioner products tend to contain much less water than shampoos and often contain a wide range of humectants, moisturizers, oils, and small amounts of proteins to improve the overall quality of the hair. Conditioners, especially those formulated for dry, coarse, or curly hair, often contain silicone-based ingredients to smooth the hair fibers.

Silicones, commonly referred to as "cones" on Internet hair forums, coat the hair shaft in a thin, breathable layer of protection that allows the strands to move freely and easily past one another. These products are easily identified by their common word endings: *-cone, -conol, -col and –xane*—and you either love them or you hate them! Silicones generally have a lighter feel on the hair than oils but can be more difficult to wash away. These ingredients are included in conditioners primarily to improve wet combing and to enhance shine—but, if silicone-based products tend to weigh your hair down, going silicone-free may be right for you.

Types of Conditioners

In Hair Care Rehab, there are four main types of conditioners:

1. Instant & cream-rinse conditioners,

2. Deep conditioners,

3. Protein reconstructors/treatments, and

4. Leave-in conditioners.

Instant & Cream-Rinse Conditioners

Instant conditioners are thin and lotionlike because of their high water content. Since the ingredients in these conditioners are often too large to penetrate the hair, they do not deep condition well. These watery products are generally best suited for those with fine or oily hair types, and are the best rinse-out conditioners to leave in. Instant conditioner formulas rinse from the hair easily and cleanly.

Cream-rinse conditioners are generally used as a final rinse, and like many instant conditioners, they are often left on the hair shaft for less than 3 to 5 minutes. Cream-rinse conditioners contain a considerable amount of shaft-smoothing ingredients such as silicones, oils, and emollients, all of which support hair detangling in those with medium to thick straight or curly hair. These conditioners also work well for protecting the hair against damage from the heat styling that may follow a shampoo-and-conditioning session.

Deep Conditioners

Deep conditioners, the focus of Detox Step 2, are wonderful because they tend to contain a concentrated mixture of both moisture and protein boosting elements. Moisture simply increases the softness and elasticity of the hair, and proteins strengthen and reinforce the hair's outer layers. Strengthening the outer layers allows the hair to hold on to the moisture it receives until the next deep-conditioning treatment. Heat is often used with deep conditioners to ensure the best penetration of moisture and adhesion of protein molecules and other cuticle-protecting substances to the hair shaft.

Although deep conditioners often contain both moisture and protein ingredients, they can be classified as either *moisture-based* or *protein-based* products. This is simply because, in most

products, one characteristic is almost always emphasized over the other. Protein-based conditioners toughen the hair and tend to have words such as "anti-breakage" or "hair repair" on the labels. Moisture-based conditioners are superb detanglers and tend to use words such as "moisturizing" or "hydrating" instead. Protein and moisture-based products must be balanced in a hair care routine to protect the hair against damage. We'll talk more in the next few pages about how you can determine which type of deep conditioner to use.

Deep conditioners may be used weekly (or every 7 to 10 days) on damaged hair, especially chemically-treated hair. Once hair regains its strength, deep-conditioning frequency then becomes a matter of personal choice. Those with relatively healthy hair may choose to deep condition weekly or every 2 to 4 weeks as needed.

Protein Reconstructors/Treatments

Protein reconstructors offer more concentrated levels of protein than other conditioners. Their main purpose is to increase the tensile strength of the hair strand. Given this hard-core focus on strength-building, reconstructors rarely provide noticeable conditioning properties and often need to be followed up with an additional moisturizing deep-conditioning treatment or a great moisturizing leave-in product to restore the hair's proper elasticity and softness. Since these treatments work deeply to penetrate and rebuild the most damaged hair shafts from within, their results are more dramatic and longer lasting than those of other conditioner products.

Much of the protein in these products has been broken down into smaller components and is the correct molecular size to be absorbed into the cuticle.

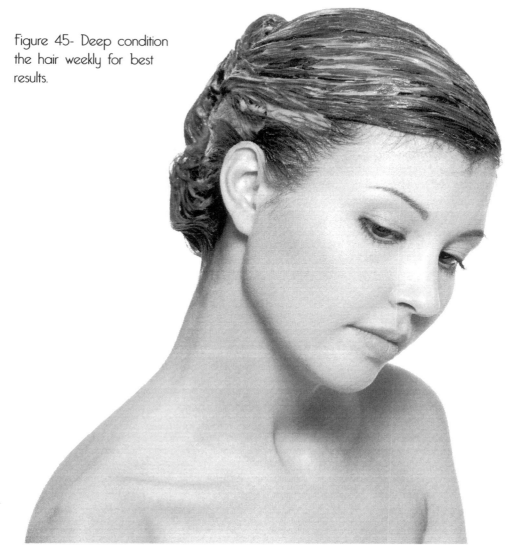

Figure 45- Deep condition the hair weekly for best results.

Leave-In Conditioners

Leave-in conditioners come in the form of both creams and liquids, and some are dually formulated as detangling products. Creamy leave-ins are best for those with thick, coarse hair, while lotions and mists often suffice for those with finer hair types. Leave-in conditioners are also excellent for those with fine to medium hair who wish to use a smoothing product for light control of their style. Mist-type leave-ins are great for touching up and reinvigorating curly and coily tresses throughout the day.

Should I Use a Moisturizing or Protein-based Deep Conditioner?

Initially, we want to focus on restoring our hair's moisture profile—that's why you should use a moisturizing deep conditioner for the first two deep conditionings. At the third conditioning (Week 3), you'll need to assess whether or not your hair needs another week of moisture, or if it's time to rotate in a protein conditioner for strength. Relying too heavily on either type of conditioner can lead to unwanted breakage problems. How will you know if you really need to switch to protein conditioning during your repair schedule? You should switch to the protein conditioner *only* if your hair meets the requirements outlined in the assessment list below. In general, here's how you can tell if you need more protein in your regimen:

Hair that needs more protein

- Is very stretchy.
- Breaks due to stretching.
- Feels weak, gummy, mushy or limp.

Hair that needs more moisture

- Does not stretch very much before breaking.
- Feels rough, tangly, dry and brittle.

To add in protein conditioning: After rinsing your shampoo, simply apply a protein conditioner or protein reconstructor product. Since reconstructors tend to make hair firmer and can leave the hair rather tangly, you may need to use a light moisturizing conditioner immediately afterward to help with detangling or to restore a bit of softness.

OPTIONAL: After deep conditioning, finish the conditioning session by rinsing the hair with an apple cider vinegar rinse (see Special Treatments, page 250) to close the cuticle and enhance your hair's shine.

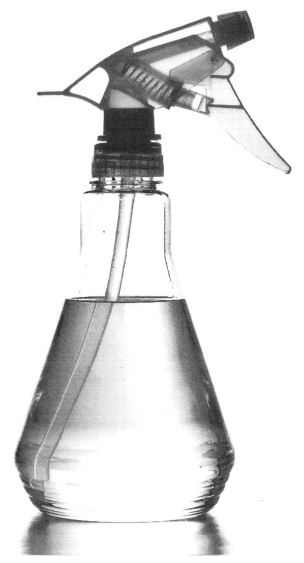

Figure 46- All hair needs adequate hydration.

Step 3: Moisturize Your Hair to Decrease Friction

Rehab R$_x$

Step 3: Moisturize your hair.
After rinsing out the conditioner in Step 2, add a layer of leave-on protection to the hair fiber. You may use a leave-in conditioner or dedicated moisturizing product—or both. If your hair is thick, dry or curly, this product should hydrate and add "slip" to your hair. If your hair is fine or oily, it should detangle while encouraging volume. Thirsty hair may require daily applications of your moisture product, while other hair types may need less frequent applications.

NOTE: If your hair is naturally oily or fine/medium textured, you may modify or skip this moisturizing step. For the finest hair types, your rinse-out conditioner may be adequate.

For a full list of product recommendations, see On the Shelf!, page 266.

Water-Based Moisturizers

Because our hair regularly exchanges moisture with the environment, moisture retention is a challenge for all hair types. In Step 3, we focus on hydrating the hair and reducing friction between the hair fibers. Moisturizers can come in the form of light sprays, creams, mousses, custards, pastes, and puddings—and many styling products fit into this category. Leave-in conditioners are actually a type of water-based moisturizer.

What's in There?

Moisturizers contain water, light emollients, humectants for attracting more moisture, gentle proteins and oils. These products do two things for the hair. They support the hair's infrastructure by replenishing internal water and other essential elements that have been lost naturally to the air and to processes such as shampooing, heat styling, chemical relaxing, perming and coloring. Next, emollients and oil ingredients restore the hair's lipid-rich outer layer to prevent the escape of this moisture back into the surrounding environment.

These products may also add volume or control and give the hair a healthy looking polish or texture. For finer hair types, these moisturizing products are tasked with hydrating the hair while building volume and fullness. Sprays, mists, foams, and ultra-light lotions work well for those with fine hair or braided hair styles. Products for thicker, drier types of hair are designed to hydrate, detangle and add weight to the hair. Lotions, creams and custards are generally best for those with thicker, coarser hair.

Depending on the formula's consistency and your hair type (thick, medium, fine), you may choose to use a leave-in conditioner product plus a second dedicated moisturizer or only one of these two products— after washing your hair. Coarser, thicker hair typically feels better with two separate moisturizing products used one after the other.

However, if your hair is a medium to ultra-fine in texture, your leave-in conditioner will very likely be enough and eliminate the need for a second water-based moisturizer product.

Moisturizers may be used daily or as needed to maintain the hair's elasticity.

NOTE: Oils and moisturizers must never be confused or used interchangeably to combat dryness. Oils work to form an impenetrable barrier so that moisture contained within a strand stays there.

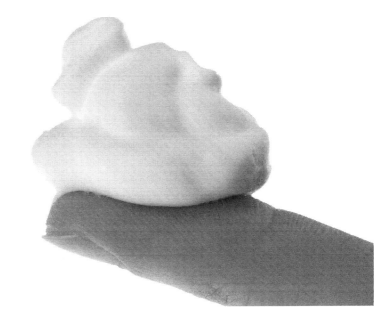

Figure 47- Foam and liquid moisturizer products are great for fine and oily hair types.

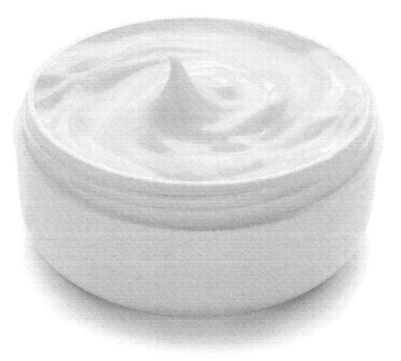

Figure 48- Cream and butter-based products work best for curly and medium to thick textured tresses.

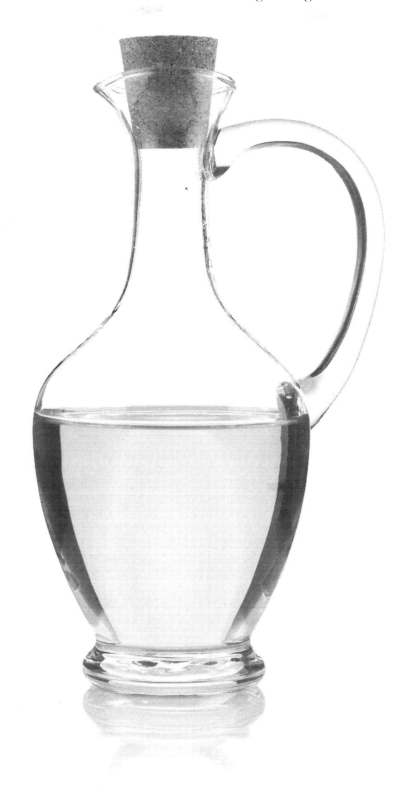

Figure 49- Oils make great sealants for moisture.

Step 4: Seal Your Hair

Rehab R$_x$

Step 4: Seal your hair.
After moisturizing your hair in Step 3, apply an oil or butter product to seal in the moisturizer. The sealing step helps to smooth the cuticle and keep the hair in a moisturized state for a longer period of time. Sealants temporarily trap in moisture. Always use oils on slightly damp/misted hair, or pair them with a water-based moisturizer to maximize your hydration benefit.

NOTE: If your hair is naturally oily or medium/fine textured, you may skip the sealing step. For the finest hair types, your rinse-out conditioner or leave-in moisturizer may be adequate moisture sealants on their own.

For a full list of product recommendations, see On the Shelf!, page 267.

Oils & Butters

If your hair is dry, super curly or thick, you are probably no stranger to the amazing world of oils and butter products. Oils and butters enhance the shine, softness, and flexibility of our hair fibers. Hair serums and polishers also fall into the oil category. These products add gloss and shine to final styles and can be used as heat protectants. Oils and butters derived from plants, flowers, seeds, and fruits are superior healthy hair care oils. They form light, semipermeable films on the exterior of the hair cuticle to help seal in moisture. Depending on their chemistry, many of these oils quickly wear off from the hair's surface or actively penetrate the hair fiber over time to provide opportunities for remoisturization of the fiber with a water-based moisturizer.

Oils as Moisturizers?

Oils are not moisturizers—they are sealants that *support* moisturization. But, the idea that basic oils, butters and serums moisturize the hair dates way back into antiquity. Lengthy debates continue in the real world and online about this very topic. Product manufacturers have not helped the issue by continuing to refer to all sorts of oils and serums as moisturizers. The confusion arises because oils and moisturizers do have some similarities. Like true moisturizers, oils, greases, and serums do

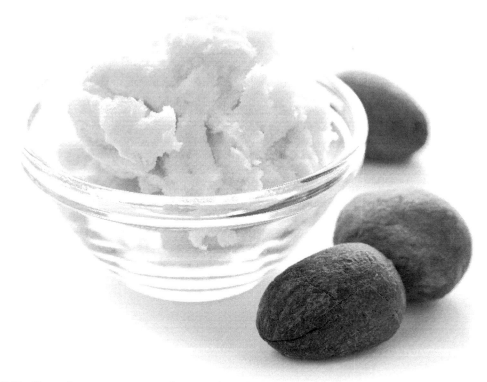

Figure 50- Shea butter is a great hair sealant for moisture.

soften, nourish, add shine, and increase the hair's pliability.

However, the old saying, *Oil and water do not mix*, certainly holds true in hair care. When oils are placed on the hair before a moisturizing product (or as a moisturizing product), they form a seal that prevents real moisture from getting into the hair. This can lead to extreme dryness over time. Oils are unable to bind to water, and hair products that contain both oils and water require special blending ingredients called emulsifiers to keep the mixture from separating. Because there can be no moisture delivery without water, water is always listed as a first ingredient in moisturizing products. For best results, always apply any oil to the hair *after* it has been properly hydrated with water or a moisturizing product.

Selecting an Oil

If you choose to use an oil product in your regimen, select one with a consistency that is appropriate for your hair type. Fine strands can clump together and be easily weighed down by some oils, while coarser hair types tend to thrive with heavier oil and butter products.

If your strands are fine and you'd like to try sealing, start off with a very small amount of a very light oil such as coconut, camellia, or jojoba. We're talking fractions or roughly a half-a-pea-sized amount of oil—tops. Be very careful to start in small increments. Remember, you can always add more oil if needed! Coconut oil is a great oil to try because it slowly migrates *into* the hair fiber.

Check out the On the Shelf! section in the back of this book for more oil and butter recommendations.

Experimentation is also key! Oils that seem to work amazingly well for some may be too greasy for others. If any amount of oil still weighs your strands down, it is okay to skip this step.

Using Oils and Butters

Remember, sealants should be applied to hair that is already moisturized. Add just a touch of oil, serum or butter to your palms and carefully warm and distribute the product in your hands by rubbing them together. Work the product into the hair from mid-shaft to the ends.

Essential Oils

Essential oils are plant-based oils with small molecules that evaporate quickly from the skin. Their watery consistency and high price for tiny volumes make sealing the hair with these oils impractical—so they are not used in Hair Care Rehab. These oils are best for scalp massage or product enhancement. (Check out the On the Shelf! section in the back of this book for essential oil recommendations.) Always consult a physician prior to trying essential oils, especially if you are a woman who is pregnant or nursing.

Using Essential Oils

Essential oils are extremely potent. They should be used only 3 to 4 drops at a time and must be diluted in a thicker oil prior to using them on the scalp skin. These thicker oils are known as "carrier" oils because they carry the essential oils and help to spread them out over a larger coverage area. Proper dilution is the key. Too much carrier oil, and you risk drowning out the benefits of your essential oil.

TIP: Misting the hair with a spray moisturizer and sealing the hair with a light coating of oil before bed is good way to keep the hair moisturized and breakage free as you toss and turn at night.

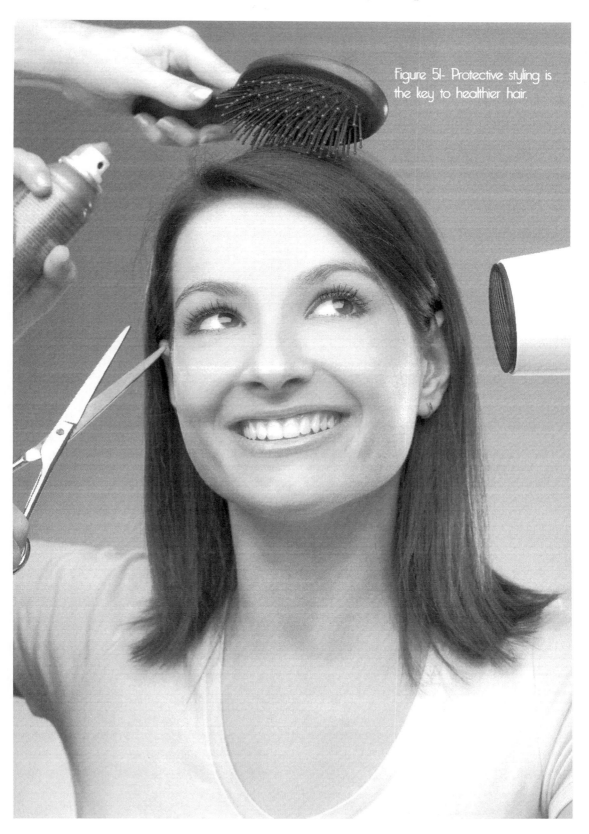

Figure 51- Protective styling is the key to healthier hair.

Step 5: Style Your Hair Protectively

If you wore your favorite sweater every single day and washed, dried and ironed it several times per week—what would it look like in a year or two? It wouldn't be pretty, that's for sure! Unfortunately, this is exactly what happens to our hair in its lifetime—and those are usually the fortunate strands that haven't been dyed, permed or bleached yet!

You hear it time and time again: The ends of our hair are the oldest parts. This is true! The ends are much more susceptible to breakage, splitting and length loss, especially if the hair is quite long. The ends of our hair strands have been through several scorching hot summers, blistering winters, and, of course, normal washing wear and tear. What can we do to preserve our hair fibers and prevent them from wearing out over time? Protective styling.

What Is Protective Styling?

Protective styling is the final step of Rehab and is basically a regimen-building technique that involves reducing overall hair manipulation. From cleansing to conditioning and general handling—everything is done with protection in mind. Here are some tips for building protection into your hair care regimen:

I. Wear Your Hair up More Often

Wearing the hair down, or out and uncontained, for a majority of the time causes the ends of the hair to fray and wear down faster. When hair is repeatedly worn down along the back (or excessively heat styled and handled), it becomes more and more necessary to trim the hair to remove those damaged, worn ends. If you wear your hair up more, you'll save and preserve the ends of your hair so that you can gain length over time. Common protective styles include an array of buns, chic ponytails, tucked ponytails, chignons, twists, braids, locs, and some weave styles. Short hair that does not yet reach the shoulders is also protective by default.

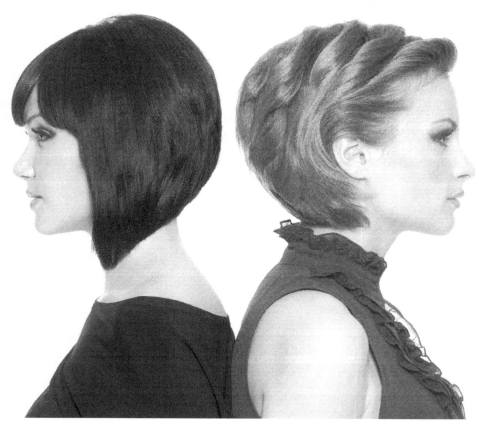

Figure 52- Short hair is naturally protective.

2. Cleanse Your Hair Protectively

Cleansing time is a great opportunity to build protection into your regimen. Carefully detangle your hair prior to washing—and wash and work in sections whenever possible. If your hair is easily manageable during the washing process, or if the hair is too short to realistically accommodate working in sections, simply keep your hair oriented downward so that water and product flows down along the hair in harmony with the natural orientation of the cuticle. Keeping your hair organized in this manner will reduce the opportunity for tangling and unnecessary breakage.

When you are cleansing your hair, ensure that your water is not too hot or too hard (mineral heavy). Hot water is very damaging to our hair,

and if your hair is color-treated, it will also fade your color quickly. Hard water also leaves invisible films on the hair that lead to dryness and breakage.

3. Detangle with Care

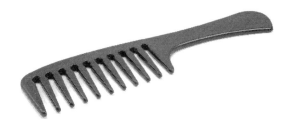

Figure 53- A large-tooth comb will reduce damage to the hair during detangling and styling.

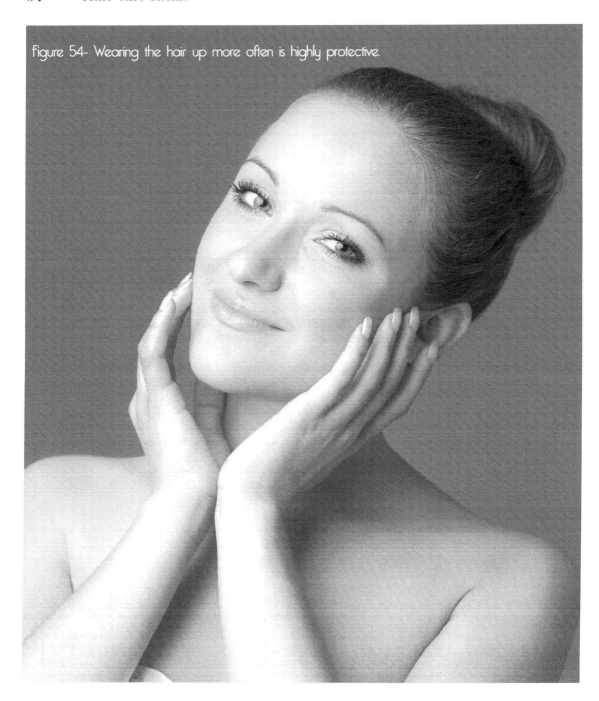

figure 54- Wearing the hair up more often is highly protective.

Combing and brushing through the hair always increases damage to the hair fiber, no matter how gently you are working. Always start at the ends of the hair and work in small sections when detangling the hair. It may also help to add a moisturizer or oil to the hair to aid in the detangling process. Slowly combine your hair as you complete the sections you've already worked on. Use your fingers to separate out the major tangles, and start from the ends of each section. Carefully and gently work your way toward the scalp with detangling.

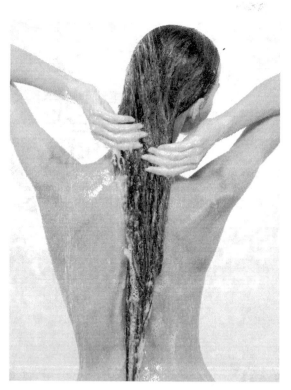

Figure 55- Great care should be taken during the cleansing phase to prevent damage.

Finger styling is a key element of protective styling the hair for everyone, especially for those with curly or textured hair types. Always begin any detangling with a thorough finger combing first, followed by a large- or wide-tooth comb.

If your hair is curly or kinky/coily, limit serious detangling efforts to wash days. Wet hair is more elastic and will move and give way to the comb more easily. However, even then, great care should be used when handling the hair in its wet state. Wet hair is naturally more fragile than dry hair.

4.   Use Heat Protectively
Heat use (other than for deep conditioning) should be limited or avoided entirely while you are trying to rehabilitate your hair. Air drying is the preferred method of hair drying for maintaining optimal hair health.

But, wait. I get it.

Let's be realistic here. You don't have time to wait for your hair to dry, especially if you are a morning hair washer, live in a cold climate, or simply don't like the way your hair dries left to its own devices. Every commonsense hair book or article tells you to avoid heat as much as possible, and I am saying that too! But, I know you. I'll issue a ban on heat styling, and only a few of you will ever have the strength and resolve to permanently say goodbye to heat styling forever! Plus, no one can deny that blow drying is fast and easy, and flat ironing can really add that extra bit of polish to a style. So, instead of telling you the horrors of regular heat use (which you probably already know, especially if you saw fit to read this book), it makes more sense for me to give tips on reducing heat damage when it is used in a hair regimen.

If you must blow dry the hair, understand that you are going to be faced with some level of hair damage in the end—especially if your hair is already dealing with some other form of hair damage. It's just part of the deal. But to reduce the chances for extra dryness, frizziness, and damage from heat styling, follow these steps:

1. After thoroughly conditioning your hair, carefully blot the hair first with a microfiber towel. Blotting is the key. Rubbing will simply cause unnecessary ruffling of the cuticle layer.

2. Apply a heat-protectant spray or cream to the hair.

3. Hold the dryer 6 to 10 inches away from your head, and direct the air down the hair shaft—not at the head.

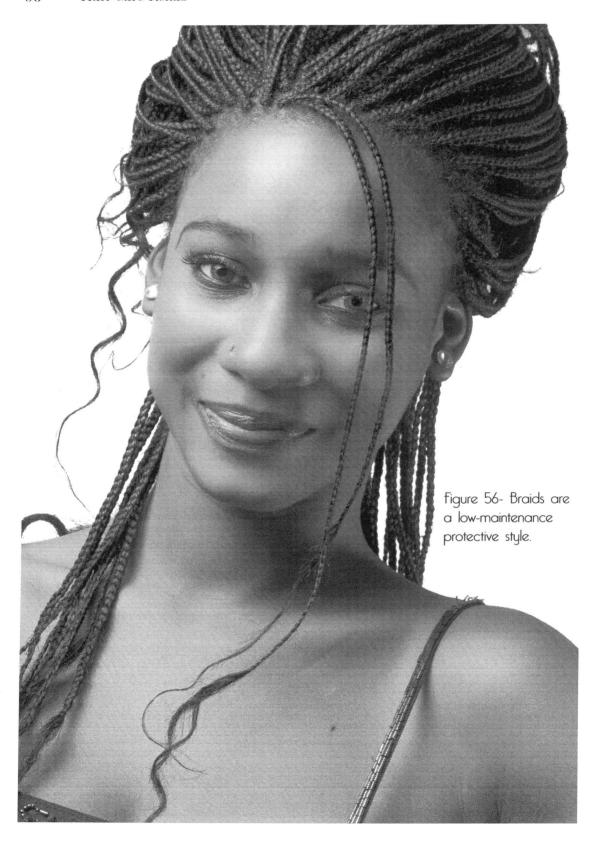

Figure 56- Braids are a low-maintenance protective style.

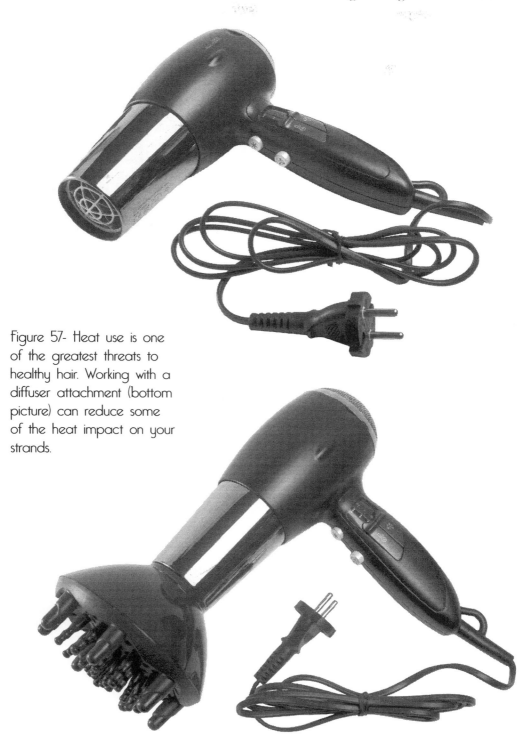

Figure 57- Heat use is one of the greatest threats to healthy hair. Working with a diffuser attachment (bottom picture) can reduce some of the heat impact on your strands.

4. Blow dry on the warmest setting while the hair is wettest, and reduce the blow dryer's heat and speed as your hair begins to dry.

Number 4 is where most of us go wrong. We either keep the heat consistent from start to finish—or start with gentle heat, and then fire it up as the hair begins to dry. It's also very tempting to think that you can start air drying your hair, and then finish up the drying with a quick blow dry. Wrong! You want to do the blowing when your hair's moisture content is the highest, and then adjust the heat downward as the moisture leaves your hair.

It sounds counterintuitive, but it's true. Our hair is most damaged from rapid heating of the hair fiber. The extra water in your hair works as a buffer against the heat. Less water = less buffer, so dried hair heats more rapidly than wet hair. Heat protectants are important because they are also a buffer against heat. These products slow the transfer of heat from your appliance to the hair. (More on this in the Heat Damage section of the Hair Repair Manual, page 186.)

Remember, heat use in general is rarely good for your hair, and some hair types can handle more heat than others. Just because your sister or friend fires up her irons daily and has amazing hair doesn't mean you'll come out the same way. It's like those people who can eat anything they want and never gain a pound! If you are serious about really getting your hair healthy, you'll have some tough decisions to make about playing with heat in your regimen. Think of heat use like alcohol consumption: A sip of wine here or there won't hurt you, but regular drinking can lead to problems down the road. Use heat (and, of course, alcohol) responsibly!

5.   Color Your Hair Protectively

If coloring is your thing, commit to coloring your hair no more than three shades lighter or darker than your natural color range. For the safest color changes, stick with rinses, semipermanent colors, and deposit-only colors such as henna (body art quality only!). These colors will not damage the cuticle or cause structural changes within the cortex. If you prefer more adventurous

coloring, have it done professionally, and ensure that you maintain a proper protein/moisture balance for your hair (Refer to Step 2). Although maintaining this balance is important for all hair types and conditions, it is absolutely essential for those with damaged or chemically-treated hair. Learning to pick up on the signs of too much usage of either protein or moisture is vital to breakage reduction and control.

6.   Reduce Chemical Use

If your hair is chemically treated in any way, stretching out the length of time between your touch-up applications will help build more protection into your hair care regimen. While this technique will not undo any damage you incur from these processes, it can still improve the overall condition of your hair when compared to chemically treating on a more rigorous schedule.

With hair coloring, you simply want to avoid taking multiple spins around the color wheel— especially if the colors you select are several shades outside of your natural color range.

7.   Slow & Steady

Finally, work slowly on your hair. Even healthy hair will break if it is manipulated too quickly from position to position. Move slowly, and give your hair the opportunity to maneuver into place. Avoid quick, short bursts of combing or brushing activity as these will certainly break both damaged and otherwise healthy strands with sheer force. This is especially true when you are using heat in conjunction with your styling tool.

Life after Rehab

After your four-week detox, you can continue with this basic repair regimen to keep your hair in great shape. Pay close attention to your protein/moisture balance to determine which conditioning regimen to follow. Hard, dry hair? Give it moisture in Step 2. Soft, stretchy, weak hair? Give it protein in Step 2.

Once your hair begins to improve, you may slowly add in minimal heat styling (no more than once or twice per week for resilient hair). Most hair types cannot handle heat more than once each week. For hair that does not respond to the four-week damage repair regimen, a trim may be in order to remove the damaged strands.

Chapter 5 Rehab Recap

And there you have it!

It may seem like a lot of information to take in—but implementing just one of the five steps today will improve your hair's condition dramatically. Improving the look and feel of hair after a damaging experience can take a few weeks of diligent moisturizing and deep conditioning to achieve. Try the Five-Step Healthy Hair Detox Regimen for four weeks, and you'll begin to notice improvement!

- You can start the hair recovery process with just five simple steps.
- Five-Step Detox Regimen Recap:

  1.) Cleanse your hair by chelating first,
  2.) Deep condition your hair with moisture and protein,
  3.) Moisturize your hair,
  4.) Seal your hair, and
  5.) Protectively style your hair.

- Important Detox Modifications:

  Step 1 (Modification)
  Beyond the initial cleansing, there will be a change from a chelating first shampoo to a more moisturizing, sulfate-free formula thereafter. If you wash your hair more than once per week, only the first shampoo in Week 1 should include the chelating shampoo— everything else should be a sulfate-free hydrating formula.

  Step 2
  The Step 2 change will involve assessing your hair to determine whether to continue on with the moisturizing deep conditioner or to change course, and introduce a protein-based deep conditioner. Again, you should only switch to the protein conditioner if your hair meets the requirements outlined in the wet-hair assessment guidelines. If you wash your hair more than once per week, then only one of these cleansings needs to include a deep-conditioning session.

Unit III:
Hair Therapy & Treatment

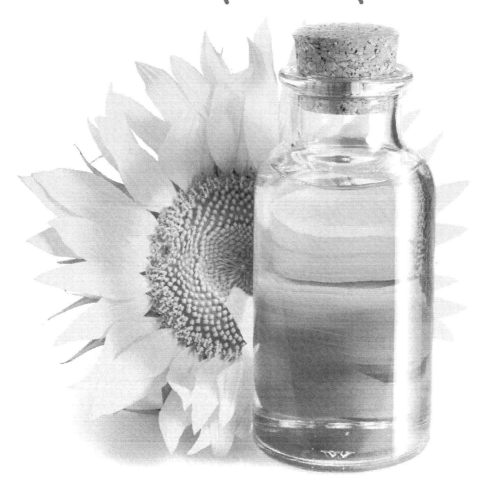

Chapter 6:

The Hair Repair Manual

Now that we've learned more about the scalp and hair, defined damage, and have reviewed some preliminary treatments that can be added to our hair repair arsenal, let's get started with addressing some common hair and scalp problems. Each rehab section includes a discussion about triggers (causes), an intervention (solutions), and avoiding relapse (prevention). Remember as you read that hair recovery and repair are always temporary hair states. *We can temporarily restore hair to a presentable and acceptable condition, but it cannot be permanently repaired.*

Now, before you venture off to rehab to find the solutions for your hair and scalp issues, bear in mind that this collection of tips and solutions is not intended to diagnose medical conditions, nor should it be substituted for medical advice. The Hair Repair Manual is not a medical treatment guide, and its tips and ideas are presented for informational purposes only. Some of the remedies and methods presented here flat out won't work for you—simple as that! You must use your best judgment and should always let your doctor know about any remedies and treatments you plan to try. Some natural remedies may interfere with traditional treatments for your condition. Remember, too, that even seemingly "natural" cures and solutions may negatively affect your health.

The Hair Repair Manual describes basic strategies that may be considered nontraditional methods. Although these types of treatments are steadily gaining popularity, it is still important to note that many of the methods have not been subjected to the same rigorous tests that traditional medical treatments have. Again, use your best judgment, and have fun experimenting!

Basic Hair & Scalp Treatment Techniques

Basic hair repair, or hair reconditioning, begins with identifying the hair problem and assigning the appropriate treatment to fix it. In this book you will learn several types of conditioning treatments. You may occasionally see these treatments referred to in the solutions to common hair and scalp problems in this book. You should experiment with them, varying your products and conditioning times to determine how best to incorporate them into your regimen.

While some of the treatments are optional, "feel-good" kinds of treatments, one in particular is key to solving nearly every hair-related issue we face.

Pre- & Post-shampoo Treatments

Pre- and post-shampoo treatments are optional treatments that are applied to the hair usually before, and sometimes after, the shampoo stage in the washing process. These treatments can be done with either warmed conditioner, oil, or a combination of both. These moisture and softness-boosting treatments help dry hair regain its suppleness and elasticity.

Pre-shampoo Treatments

Pre-shampoo treatments are usually done 20 to 30 minutes prior to cleansing the hair or as an overnight treatment before the wash. In a pre-shampoo treatment, the hair is simply covered in conditioner, which is then allowed to sit on the hair undisturbed for about 15 to 20 minutes. The hair is then rinsed and shampooed. These treatments can be performed on dry or damp hair. Some people find that doing pre-shampoo treatments on dampened hair allows the fiber to absorb moisture-boosting products with greater ease. Others find that their dry hair receives the treatments better. You will need to experiment to discover what works best for you.

Post-shampoo Treatments

Unlike pre-shampoo treatments, post-shampoo treatments follow the shampoo stage rather than precede it. Hot-oil treatments typically fall into the post-shampoo category. Increasingly, however, many people are finding utility in applying hot-oil treatments at the pre-shampoo stage as well. Water-based products such as conditioners work best for penetration into the hair fiber, while oils are better cuticle-nourishing products.

Deep Conditioning Treatments

Another type of special conditioning treatment is the deep-conditioning treatment. This treatment involves a concentrated conditioner product that follows the application of a shampoo. Deep conditioners should be used weekly on damaged hair, and are a part of the hair repair strategy for nearly every hair and scalp condition covered in this book. Those with relatively healthy hair may choose to deep condition weekly, or every 2 to 4 weeks as needed, for 10 to 15 minutes.

Rinses

A final type of hair treatment is the conditioning rinse. Rinses are treatments that follow the conditioning stage of the cleansing process. Like our healthy hair, these treatments are usually acidic in nature (pH of less than 7). These low pH products help support proper closure of the hair cuticle and effective pH balancing of the scalp environment.

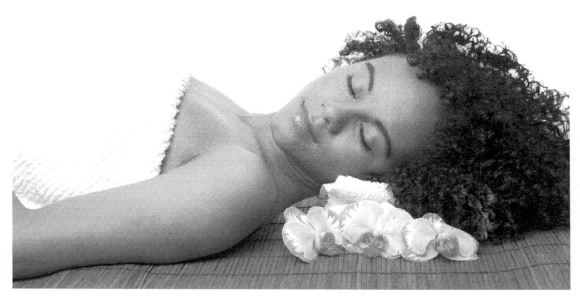

Figure 58- The Hair Repair Manual will answer over 30 of your common hair care issues.

Alopecia (Hair Loss)

Hair loss is a normal part of the human hair life cycle, but parting with even a few strands of hair can be a devastating experience for both men and women. Problems with hair loss often occur as we age or as the body is exposed to traumatic events. For some, profuse hair loss begins early and without provocation. The gradual, progressive loss of hair from the human scalp is a dermatologic condition known as alopecia. The tips in this section will help you understand alopecia and learn how to come to terms with this condition.

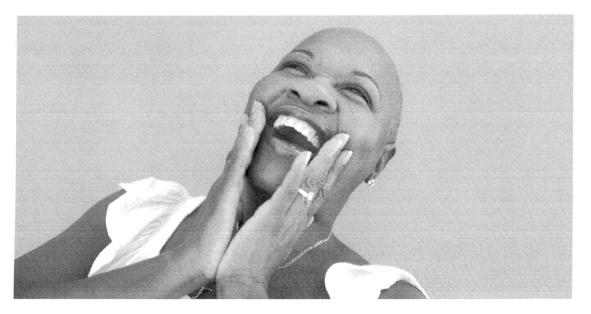

Signs & Symptoms

- Severe hair thinning, either concentrated or diffuse.
- One or more patches of hair loss.

Causes & Triggers
Alopecia can affect anyone at any time. Different forms of alopecia have their own proposed causes and triggers.

Traction Alopecia
Traction alopecia is a form of hair loss brought on by stress to the hair follicles. This form of alopecia is most often caused by tight hairstyles that place tension on delicate hair follicles. Over time, the hair follicles are stressed to the point that they begin to shrink and produce finer and finer hair strands. Eventually, no hair is produced at all from these follicles. Traction alopecia can occur with any hair type that is placed in

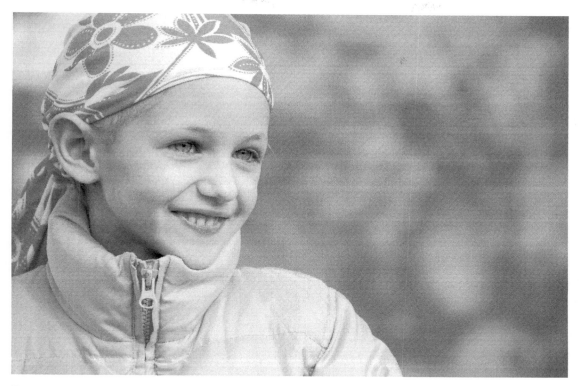

Figure 59- Alopecia can affect people of all ages.

tension-bearing styles such as tight ponytails, poorly fitting wigs, hair buns, braids or tight headwraps and scarves on a regular basis. This form of alopecia is especially common among those with textured hair types as tension is often placed around the delicate hairline area to create smooth, neat styles.

Androgenic Alopecia
Androgenic alopecia is an inherited form of hair loss that is thought to be caused by sensitivity to certain hormones in the body.

Alopecia Areata
Alopecia areata is a form of hair loss that occurs when the immune system suddenly mounts an attack against the hair follicles. Alopecia areata often occurs without warning, and hair loss is typically spotty and random. For many sufferers, the condition usually resolves itself, and hair growth resumes without treatment in about a

year's time. For others, however, the condition may be permanent. This form of hair loss tends to come and go, and the larger the affected area and the longer the baldness lasts, the less likely the chances for hair regrowth.

Alopecia Totalis/Universalis
In alopecia totalis, alopecia areata expands to include the entire head of hair. In alopecia universalis, the entire body loses its hair.

Cancer-Therapy Related Alopecia
If you've been diagnosed with cancer, it is very likely that you will have to deal with the prospect of treatment-related hair loss. Chemotherapy medications and radiation treatments can trigger alopecia. Contrary to popular belief, however, not all cancer therapies trigger hair loss. Your doctor will be able to give you an idea about what you can expect from your particular treatment. Unfortunately, as of this writing, there are not

yet any 100 percent–effective, advance treatments for preventing the hair loss brought on by cancer therapies.

Chemotherapy

Chemotherapy treatments target the body's rapidly growing cells in an attempt to destroy fast-growing cancerous cells. But since hair cells are also some of the fastest-replicating cells in the body, chemotherapy has a devastating effect on them. The degree of hair loss that you can expect with these therapies depends on the dose and combination of chemotherapy drugs or radiation received. Some chemotherapy drugs do not cause hair loss in patients. When hair loss does occur, it may affect the entire body or just certain parts of the body such as the eyebrows and lashes. The length of time spent in treatment also plays a role in determining whether hair loss will be limited to thinning or evolve into total hair loss.

If hair loss does occur, the hair typically begins to fall out one to three weeks after the first chemotherapy treatment. Chemotherapy drugs are potent and act fast on all quickly dividing cells in the body. Hair may often come out in large clumps with very little manipulation or pulling. The fallen hair that accompanies chemotherapy is also different from regular shed hairs because many of the strands do not contain the telltale white "root" tip on the scalp end of the hair. This white tip is missing because the chemo treatment does not give the hair follicles time to cycle through their natural growing and shedding phases.

Chemotherapy hair loss is almost always temporary. Lost hair may begin growing back during treatment, or three to six months after the final treatment course. Do note that once treatments such as chemo or other medications are discontinued, the hair that returns may be of a different texture or color than the pretreatment hair.

Radiation Therapy

Radiation-therapy-induced alopecia, unlike hair loss due to chemotherapy, is often irreversible and only affects hair in the area receiving the treatment. For example, radiation treatments for breast cancer may involve some radiation dosing to the underarm area during the course of treatment. In this case, underarm hair may begin to fall out. When hair does return following radiation treatment, the new hair usually returns three to six months after treatment ends and is often sparse and patchy.

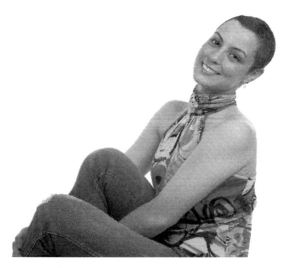

Figure 60- Hair regrowth is possible with some forms of alopecia.

When It's Time to See Your Doctor
If you notice hair thinning or unusual patchy hair loss on your scalp, eyelashes, eyebrows, underarms or other areas see a licensed dermatologist for an official diagnosis. Your dermatologist will likely perform blood tests and/or a scalp analysis to determine a suitable treatment for your situation.

Intervention & Preventing Relapse

With alopecia, intervention and prevention can be a hit-or- miss process because modern medicine is yet to produce a foolproof method for combatting it. Some therapies may simply not work, in some cases. In situations in which alopecia is complete, even fewer options exist. Traction alopecia is by far the easiest to cure since it is brought on by self-induced, physical damage. Simply removing the physically damaging factor will help this type of alopecia if follicle miniaturization (shrinking) has not yet occurred. Although most other types of alopecia are permanent, a few therapies may help.

Cold Therapy

Saving hair before it is lost is one way to deal with alopecia. One method that is popular with cancer patients in Europe involves "shocking" the hair follicles with cold therapy. In this treatment, the scalp is covered with a special cap or hood that is filled with cold water—or simple ice packs—to stun the hair follicles just before the chemo drugs are administered. The goal is to prevent the drug from interfering with the normal function of the follicle. Since the scalp follicles and cells do not receive the full chemo treatment, much less hair is lost; however, cold therapy may also prevent chemotherapy drugs from reaching potentially cancerous cells in the scalp skin.

Cortisone Injections

Cortisone is the most common treatment for alopecia. This steroid is typically injected directly into several locations within the alopecia site with a small needle. Pain is usually minimal, and hair typically begins to regrow within a month.

Cortisone Pills

Cortisone pills are usually more effective at encouraging hair regrowth than direct cortisone injections. Pills are often used for treating hair loss that includes a considerable amount of scalp hair. Prolonged use of cortisone pills can possibly lead to other health complications, so these medications should only be taken under the care of a licensed medical professional.

Minoxidil

Minoxidil applied directly to the affected skin region is another popular treatment for alopecia. This treatment comes in liquid, foam or shampoo forms and works best for those with small patches of alopecia (alopecia areata). Treatment must be continued to prevent hair loss from reoccurring. Hair loss usually returns within a few months of ending treatment.

Anthralin Cream/Ointment

Anthralin is a tarlike cream or ointment that is applied to bare skin and works in a timed-release fashion. Since it can be irritating and tends to stain the skin, it is usually only applied briefly (usually for less than an hour) and then rinsed away. The active ingredient is slowly released over time to help reduce possible skin irritation. Used primarily for the treatment of psoriasis, it is often also used to treat alopecia areata. Hair regrowth usually occurs in two to three months.

Basic Hair Breakage

Has your hair literally reached its *breaking point*? Are you sweeping up piles and piles of hair from your bathroom floor? Clogging your shower drains? Wiping up hair from the sink? When hairs have decided to give up and simply break off rather than risk another day on top of your head, something has got to give! Hair breakage occurs when there is a net imbalance between protein and moisture in the hair fiber or when hair has simply been subjected to intense physical strain. Moisture deficiency is the leading cause of hair breakage. The tips in this section will help you get basic hair breakage issues under control once and for all!

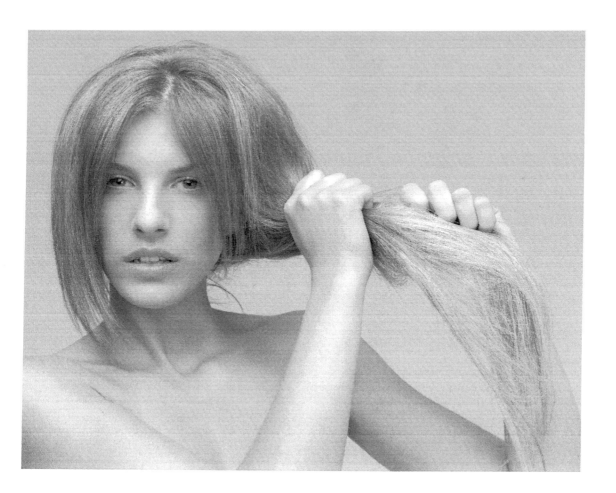

Signs & Symptoms

Hair breakage is easy to identify. Common signs and symptoms include:

- Short, broken hair strands on the floor, bathroom sink, or on clothing.
- Weak, gummy, limp hair.
- Rough, dry hair.
- Wispy, flyaway hair.
- Split ends.
- Dull, lackluster hair.

Hair breakage is the most advanced degree of hair damage we encounter. Before a strand ever reaches its breaking point, it has already lost several layers of cuticle, either from styling processes or from normal wear and tear. Where cuticle has not been lost, it has been severely lifted or cracked. Typically, hair in this distressed state has also been stretched out of shape and is well beyond its normal elastic threshold.

Causes & Triggers

The primary causes of hair breakage are simply

- Lack of moisture in the strand.
- Lack of protein in the strand.
- Overhandling and physical trauma.

While breakage can occur when the hair is handled roughly, most breakage cases can be traced back to improper protein and moisture balancing. Hairstyling techniques such as blow drying, flat ironing, thermal straightening, or hot curling can deplete moisture levels deep within the hair fiber. Processes such as permanent coloring, highlighting, perming, and chemical relaxing can deplete the hair's natural protein stores.

Our hair care products provide us with the temporary protein and moisture that we need to have strong, healthy hair fibers. But poor product choices may also push a protein or moisture deficiency into overdrive, leading to more hair breakage. When we overuse protein products such as hair repair masks, reconstructing products, and gels (when our hair needs more moisture) or splurge on moisturizing products (when our hair needs more protein), our hair always responds with additional breakage. This is why we must carefully assess and balance the protein and moisture aspects of our hair care regimens.

Many people think their hair's moisture needs are already being met, but very few of us use adequate moisture in our hair care regimens. Water and water-based products are the only true sources of moisture for our hair. Other commonly touted sources of moisture, including various oils or butters, are not sources of moisture; they are *moisture support*. They create a barrier to trap moisture in the hair, which enhances moisturization. They are not, however, the moisture source.

Without a doubt, moisture deficiency is the leading cause of hair breakage, but other stressors can weaken hair shafts to the point of breakage as well. Brushing or combing the hair too often, leaving in extensions for too long, or using improper hair tools for the job (i.e., a fine-tooth comb on extremely thick, curly strands) can lead to breakage.

When It's Time to See Your Doctor

Hair breakage is usually a simple problem that can be solved by just refocusing a hair care product regimen or reducing overall hair manipulation. If your breakage levels suddenly increase or you experience excessive shedding (from the root), along with other symptoms, consult a dermatologist.

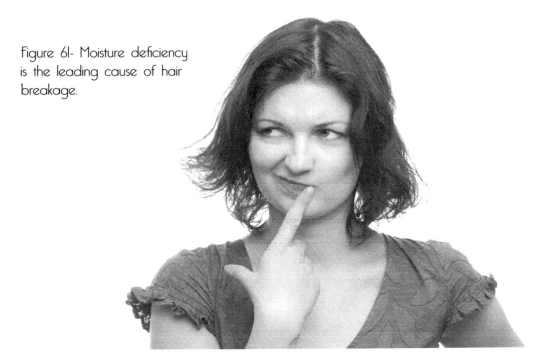

Figure 61- Moisture deficiency is the leading cause of hair breakage.

Intervention & Preventing Relapse
Perform a Wet-Hair Assessment

If you are battling with hair breakage, determining the cause and the required product solutions to stop the breakage is as simple as touching or combing through your hair while it is wet. Wet hair is the best type of hair to examine if you want to determine whether your personal protein- or moisture- balancing requirements are being properly met.

But why *wet* hair?

Wet hair excellently demonstrates our hair's basic properties of elasticity, porosity, and strength. We can judge our hair's condition as it relates to elasticity, porosity, and strength just from how it moves and behaves when it is wet. This is why cleansing and conditioning at least weekly are strongly recommended. Aside from cleanliness, you need this wash time each week to get in touch with your hair and understand what its needs are.

A wet-hair assessment should be performed every time you wash your hair. Wet hair should feel soft yet strong and should not break unless there is serious stress placed on it through detangling, arranging, or styling. If breakage *does* occur during your wet-hair assessment, the way the hair breaks under these conditions will give you a sure indication of whether more moisture or protein is required to regain the proper balance. If you are ever unsure about which treatment your hair needs to maintain its balance, clarify the hair and go with a moisturizing product plan.

Regimen-Building Tip

Always start off with a more moisture-friendly regimen before you incorporate any protein aspects. The reason is that many of us (before we enter Hair Care Rehab!) have naturally moisture-deficient hair care routines—especially those with no real regimen at all.

Wet-Hair Assessment

Balanced	Your wet hair feels strong, stretches slightly and returns to its original length with no breakage.

You Need → More Moisture   *If . . .*

More Moisture	Your wet hair feels rough, hard and tangly. Hair does not stretch much before breaking.

You Need → More Protein   *If . . .*

More Protein	If your wet hair feels weak, gummy and limp. Hair stretches and stretches before breaking.

Deep Condition

Deep conditioning is essential for fighting breakage and restoring the hair. Simply deep condition your hair for 10 to 15 minutes with the moisture- or protein-based conditioner product that you need to restore your hair's balance. Remember, heat enhances the conditioning benefits of conditioners by improving the "staying power" of most products. Always rinse conditioners with cool water.

Put Your Hair Away

To greatly reduce hair breakage, consider putting your hair up for a while. Styles like sleek buns, messy buns, carefully tucked ponytails, chignons, twists, and braids can give your hair a break without literally causing you breakage.

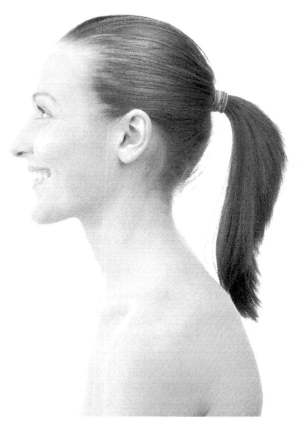

Figure 62- A low-maintenance hairstyling routine will reduce hair breakage.

Burns (Appliances)

You should have been out the door ten minutes ago—but here you are standing with one shoe on and a curling iron wrapped around your half-dried hair. You're thinking about that huge presentation you're giving today, your phone bill which is about to be past due, and why that charming guy from last weekend hasn't called you back when the curling iron suddenly slips. Ouch! Appliance burns can occur anywhere on the body—on your face, neck, ears, chest, and legs—when heat-styling tools accidentally slip, fall or get too close to skin during regular use. Fortunately for us, most appliance burns are simple burns and are easy to treat. The tips in this section can be used to soothe all types of burns.

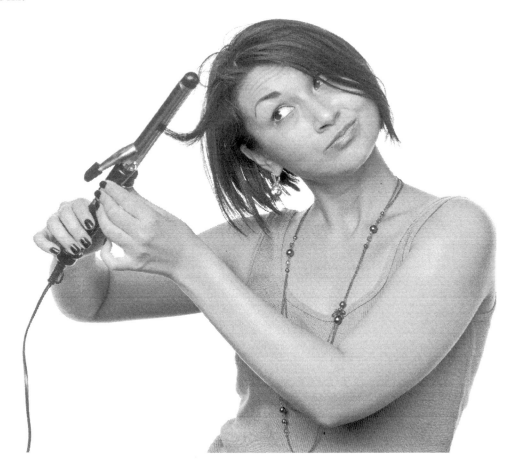

Signs & Symptoms

Many of us have not-so-fond memories of our first forehead burn from trying to curl bangs as a teenager, or mom getting too close to an ear with her flatiron or pressing comb! Then there are the newer marvels of modern hair care such as hair steamers and other steam-releasing appliances that can easily result in burns to unsuspecting users. Common signs and symptoms include:

- Red, inflamed skin.
- Swelling, possible blistering.
- Pain/discomfort.
- Scabbing in the final stage.

Causes & Triggers

Appliance burns occur when heat-styling tools are used improperly or accidently slip during normal use. These burns are usually superficial and take less than a week or two to heal.

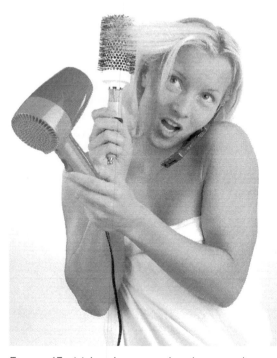

Figure 63- Multitasking can lead to appliance burns.

Intervention & Preventing Relapse

Cool Towel Compress

Immediately after your burn, cool your skin! Combating burns with cold temperatures is an age-old remedy for small burns. Simply soak a washcloth in cool water. (Milk will also work.) Wring out the excess liquid, and apply the cool towel carefully to the burned area for fast relief. If your burn is on your hand, wrist, leg, or other body part that can be placed under a running tap, expose the burn to cool running water (at low pressure) for 5 to 10 minutes to help lessen the pain. Ice-cold, freezing water should be avoided because this can actually irritate the burned skin.

Aloe Vera Therapy

One home remedy that may help your burn is aloe vera gel. The coolness of this plant-derived product helps to soothe the skin. Aloe vera gel

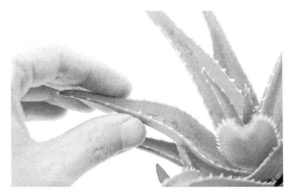

Figure 64- Aloe vera has been used for centuries to soothe burns.

also speeds the healing process and facilitates better skin-cell regeneration. Apply 100 percent aloe vera gel to the burn 3 to 4 times a day. Be sure that any bottled gel you apply does not contain additives such as alcohol, which can further irritate the skin. Keep air flow to the burn as open as possible to speed healing.

Cucumber!

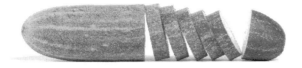

Figure 65- The cooling effects of cucumbers are perfect for temporary burn relief.

Try placing a slice of cucumber on your burn. Not only is this veggie a popular remedy in spas for puffy eyes and dark circles, this super-cool plant will also help reduce the sting and itchiness of your burn. Some have even found that a chilled potato or onion slice will do the trick as well.

Slow Down!
This one is pretty obvious, but slow it down! Burns almost always happen when you're running late or rushing to get your hair styled. If you are working with fragile areas near the nape of the neck or ears, use smaller sections or smaller styling tools to catch the small pieces. Larger sections and big tools are clunky and less precise, so they can easily result in a burn.

Keep Your Work Area Organized
If you've got a maze of cords around your bathroom sink, you've got a burn accident waiting to happen! Work with one heat-styling tool at a time. If you've got two appliances plugged into the same wall outlet together, cords can become so entangled that, when you lift up one hot appliance, the other one comes up right along with it!

Keep Heat Tools on Hard, Flat Surfaces
This advice sounds reasonable enough, but you'd be surprised by the number of appliance-burn victims who placed their irons on their beds, on top of a stack of magazines or in some other unsteady area! Keep your appliances on firm, solid surfaces.

Keep Your Distance
Avoid bringing heat appliances such as curling irons near the scalp when your roots are damp or sprayed with product. On damp hair, the appliance can create steam and burn the scalp without the appliance ever directly touching it.

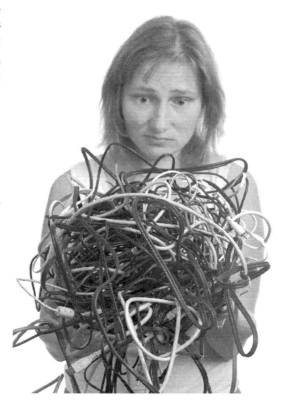

Figure 66- Keeping your work area organized will prevent many hair mistakes.

Chemical Burns

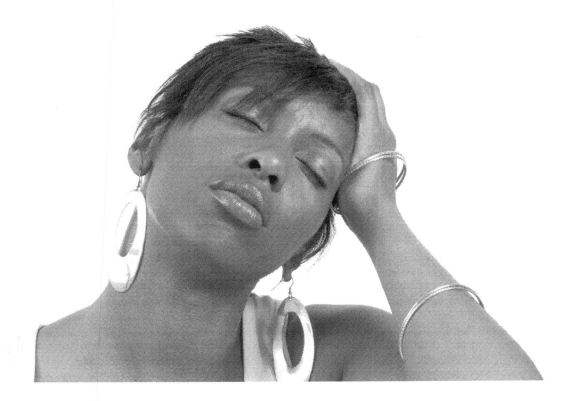

You are sitting in your stylist's chair, and all of a sudden you begin to feel that telltale tingle on your scalp, ear, or forehead that tells you that your routine color or chemical-straightening service is about to head downhill fast. With your scalp still tingling, the stylist rinses the product from your hair, but you still feel the tenderness that you know could only come from a chemical burn in the making. Once your hair is fully dried, and the dust settles, the obvious is confirmed: You've been burned. Redness, tenderness, and perhaps even a scab forms in the coming days with strands of your own hair fused in it. If it is really bad, you may experience hair loss in the affected region. If a chemical burn does happen to you, don't fret! The tips in this section, used with your doctor's approval, will help get your scalp in working order once again!

Signs & Symptoms

Burns should never be considered a normal part of the hair-styling process, and a proper strand test before chemical treatment will reveal possible sensitivities that could lead to burning. Common burn symptoms include:

- Red, inflamed skin.
- Swelling, possible blistering.
- Pain/discomfort.
- Scabbing in the final stage.

Causes & Triggers

Chemical burns are the direct result of improper chemical-product application or skin sensitivity to hair-product ingredients. These burns are usually first- and second-degree burns and can take anywhere from three days to three weeks to heal, depending on the burn. These burns happen when

- The chemical formula is too strong or not suited for your skin.
- You have an allergy or sensitivity to the chemical being used.
- The scalp is exposed to chemicals for an extended period of time.
- The scalp is irritated from scratching or other trauma prior to product application.
- The stylist employs inadequate scalp-basing and protection techniques during chemical treatments.

Intervention & Preventing Relapse

Whenever possible, chemical services should be left to professionals and experienced individuals. Always report any burning or tingling you experience during your salon visit to your stylist immediately, so that he/she may remove the product properly. If you are applying the chemical product on your own, always seek medical attention immediately if you suspect a burn.

When It's Time to See Your Doctor

Chemical burns and other burns in hair care are considered first-degree when there is only redness and tenderness and second-degree when there is watery discharge or oozing. Always watch for signs of infection such as odors, pus, and swollen lymph glands. If your burn does not seem to get better with the remedies suggested in *Hair Care Rehab*, or if you notice swollen lymph glands in the neck, please seek medical attention immediately.

The following remedies may also provide you relief:

Aloe Vera Therapy

This home remedy (also described in the appliance burns section (page 113) works well for chemical burns. Be sure to use 100 percent aloe vera gel because common additives such as alcohol and other irritants in some commercial brands can make burns worse. Apply the treatment to your burn 3 to 4 times a day.

Conditioner Treatment

Some people find that deep conditioning the hair and scalp works well to aid healing of larger burns and multiple burns that are not grouped together on the scalp. The conditioning process soothes affected areas of the scalp, and each application helps soften and loosen the scabby areas. If you've been burned by a chemical product, it is important that you avoid picking or peeling your blisters or scabs as this can lead to infection and scarring.

Tea Therapy

Black or green tea leaves contain tannic acid, an ingredient that has been used for many years to treat surface burns on the skin. Place two or

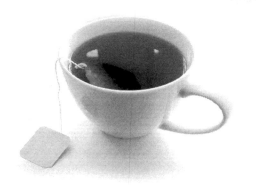

Figure 67- Tea is a quick home remedy for burns.

three tea bags in boiling water, and steep until dark. Allow the liquid to cool. Simply apply the cooled liquid to the affected area several times per day using a cotton ball.

Pre-shampoo Oatmeal Scalp Mask

Oatmeal has been used for centuries to soothe irritated skin and has soothing effects on burned skin as well. To prepare the oatmeal mask, simply combine 1 cup quick oats, ½ cup fresh milk (or water), ½ cup olive oil, and a tablespoon of honey for moisture. Gently detangle your hair, taking care not to scratch the scalp, and apply the thick oatmeal paste to the scalp. Cover with a plastic shower cap and allow the mask to remain on the hair for 20 minutes. Rinse and follow with a sulfate-free shampoo and conditioning.

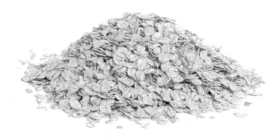

Figure 68- Oatmeal has a soothing effect on the skin

Safety First!

Prevention, of course, is the best medicine for burns—especially for chemical burns. Before beginning any chemical treatment, always read and follow the manufacturer's instructions on the products to be used, even if you have used them before with no problems. This often includes conducting a "patch test" for sensitivity prior to each and every service. Product ingredients or instructions for use may have changed since your last use of the product, so it's important not to skip this precaution.

Reduce Scalp Irritation

Avoid scratching the scalp prior to applying chemicals to the hair. Scalp irritation or breaks and vulnerabilities in the skin always lead to burns. Avoid brushing or applying heavy force to your scalp as you part it—especially around the fragile hairline.

Keeping the scalp dry before applying chemicals is another way to avoid unnecessary burning. Avoid washing hair or participating in a high-perspiration activity the day prior to chemical treatment. A freshly washed scalp is sensitive and highly susceptible to burning without its natural oils there for protection.

Be Smart about Processing Times

Process your hair for the manufacturer's suggested time for your hair type. Even a few moments beyond the suggested time could result in a burned scalp and lifeless overprocessed hair. Rinse and/or neutralize your hair thoroughly to remove all traces of the chemical product from your hair and scalp.

Lift Your Head

If you are visiting a stylist, be sure to lift your head at the shampoo bowl as your chemical treatment is being rinsed. Oftentimes, the

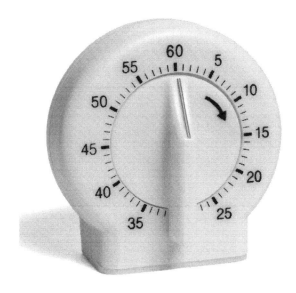

Figure 69- Keep an eye on the clock when you are working with chemicals.

uncomfortable angle of the bowl may make us want to rest our heads and necks on the rim for relief, but this can lead to overprocessing and chemical burns in the nape area. Make sure this area is rinsed thoroughly.

Chemical-Relaxing Precautions
Protect the Scalp
If you will be chemically straightening the hair, apply a thick layer of petroleum jelly or grease to the hair and scalp to protect them from the harsh relaxer chemicals. By increasing the thickness of the petroleum barrier, harsh chemicals are less likely to damage the hair and scalp. Let your stylist know if you are susceptible to burning, and inform him/her immediately if you begin to feel the tingle that often precedes full-scale burning.

Neutralize Properly
For those who undergo chemical relaxing to straighten their hair, thoroughly rinse all traces of the relaxer product from the hair. Then, neutralize all traces of relaxer that may still remain behind on your scalp with a neutralizing shampoo. This is critical. Allow your neutralizer to sit on your hair and scalp undisturbed for 3 to 5 minutes before rinsing. This will give the neutralizer a chance to bring your scalp's pH down, so that the relaxer cannot continue to work on the skin.

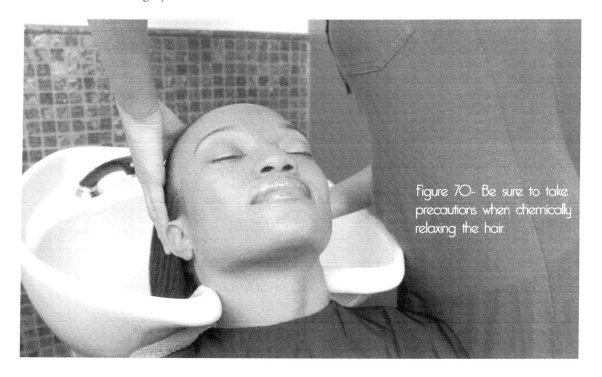

Figure 70- Be sure to take precautions when chemically relaxing the hair.

Chlorine & Pool Water Damage

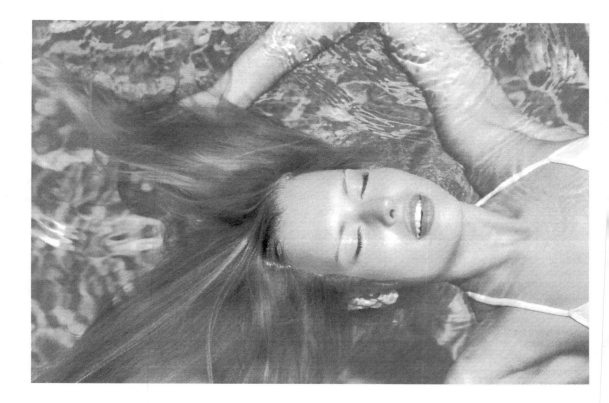

Summertime can be really hard on our hair, and those of us who swim regularly (more than once a week) know it firsthand. Chlorine from swimming pools can be so drying to our hair that even those of us who only spend a few hours here and there at the pool can feel the negative effects. (Just look at what it does to swimsuits!) Chlorine is necessary to prevent our swimming pools from becoming breeding grounds for bacteria and germs. But if our hair is left unprotected, chlorinated water can lead to dry, rough, breaking, tangly, discolored hair—especially for those with already weak, porous, chemically treated hair. The tips in this section will help you protect your hair from chlorine damage.

Signs & Symptoms
- Dry, parched, tangly hair.
- Color changes (greenish tint on light-colored strands).
- Hair breakage.

Causes & Triggers
Concentrated chlorine is great for keeping up the hygiene of pools, but it can really destroy our hair even with limited exposure. Chlorine wipes out the hair's natural oils whose job it is to keep our hair soft, manageable and flexible. With natural oils out of the picture, the hair shaft becomes more vulnerable to cracking and splitting. Chlorinated water is also responsible for the "green hair" problem that some blondes and those with lighter hair experience after swimming (see Green Hair, page 172). The higher the concentration of chlorine and the longer the exposure to the chlorinated water, the more damage you can expect.

Intervention & Preventing Relapse
Detangle Your Hair before Swimming
To prevent excessive tangling, avoid swimming with the hair loose or uncontained. Loose hair is asking for tangles, so either wear a swim cap or gather the hair into a bun or ponytail before getting into the water. If you won't be wearing a swim cap, detangle the hair before arranging it into your "contained style" because dry tangled hair = wet super-tangled hair! Proper detangling and gathering of the hair will prevent knotting that can lock in once cuticles are wet and frazzled by the pool water.

Prep Your Hair First
Never get into a pool with dry hair. If you are wearing a swimming cap, this won't be an issue, but if your hair is exposed, you'll want to drench your hair in fresh water before you ever hop into the pool. Why? Because hair can only take in so much water. If the water your hair absorbs is

fresh water, then very little chlorinated water will get in. You can also create an additional layer of protection for your hair by adding a light coating of conditioner before jumping into the pool.

Detangle Your Hair After Swimming
If you have access to an outdoor shower or rinse-off station, carefully rinse and detangle your hair with your fingers using a downward motion immediately after exiting the pool. Carefully detangling the hair after swimming will prevent matting that can occur once the hair begins to dry.

Chelate Your Hair
Chelating your hair will help to remove stubborn chlorine deposits that may affect the hair after swimming. Chelating shampoos remove dulling deposits that can lead to dryness and breakage of the hair. (See Rehab Step 1 for more on chelating shampoos.)

Reconstruct with Protein
Because chlorine can disturb the hair's protein bonds, protein reconstructors are perfect for post-swimming upkeep. These conditioners will smooth the cuticle and give the hair an added layer of strength and protection.

Deep Condition with Moisture
After reconstructing the hair with protein, deep condition the hair with a moisturizing conditioner for 10 to 15 minutes with heat to restore your hair's pliability and replenish some of the moisture lost to the reconstructing process.

Reduce Heat as Much as Possible
To really give the hair life after swimming, always air dry when you can or use diffused heat. Heat and chlorine do not mix—and the hair will always feel weak and dry when the two are combined.

Color Fading

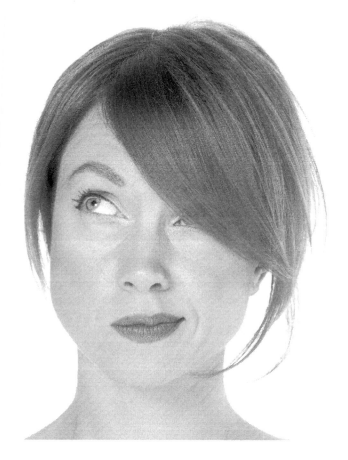

Whether it's your favorite shirt or your beautiful new hair color, no one really likes to deal with color fading. Honestly, who likes to see their hard work circling its way down the drain? While all hair colors fade with time, and no color can remain as true as it was on Day 1, it can be especially nerve-wracking if you've paid top dollar to have your hair colored by a color specialist, only to have the color fade a week later! Whether you've paid nearly the equivalent of your rent or mortgage to get your color—or just decided to work your color magic for a few dollars at home, the tips in this chapter can help preserve your hair color for longer!

Signs & Symptoms

- Dull, lackluster hair color.
- Brassy-colored hair.
- Dry hair.

Causes & Triggers

Hair-color fading can be triggered by any hairstyling process that causes the pigments deposited on the hair to leach from the fiber. Things like heat styling and simply washing the hair are primary color-fading culprits. Color fade is especially problematic with deposit-only colors such as rinses and other temporary colors. They fade faster because they sit on the outside of the hair strand. Permanent hair colors are deposited deeper into the strand, and so color fading tends to occur more slowly.

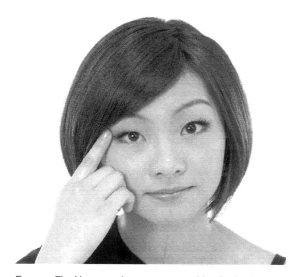

Figure 71- Heat styling can quickly fade hair colors.

Intervention & Preventing Relapse
Water Is the Enemy
Okay, maybe that's a little harsh—but it's true if you are trying to preserve your color. While water is typically a great ally in healthy hair care, it is a relative enemy to color-treated tresses. Water slowly rinses color pigments from the hair with each session, no matter which type of hair color you have used (i.e., permanent, semipermanent, or temporary). If daily washing is your thing, you might consider skipping a day or two between shampooings. For best results, allow your new hair color to settle for at least a day or two before shampooing and conditioning again.

Shampooing and conditioning your hair in hard water (or water that is partially chlorinated) will also strip your hair color. Hard water loads the hair fiber down with metal ions and scale that can quickly evaporate your shine and vibrancy—not to mention dry out your hair to a crisp! If your water is hard, or if you are a regular swimmer, consider purchasing a chelating shampoo for regular color maintenance. For longer-term results, a good water filter (although expensive) may buy you several more weeks of vibrant hair color.

Cool It Down!
While water has the power to take the *umph* out of your new color all on its own, the situation is worse if the water is hot. Hot water also encourages color release! Keep your water warm to tepid for hair washing. Shampooing your hair in hot water not only removes color faster, but it is also stressful to hair in general. Regular hot-oil treatments or other treatments that warm the hair, including long, heated deep conditioning, can have similar color-fading effects. After conditioning the hair, do a final rinse in the coldest water you can stand. This final rinse will seal the cuticle and impart amazing shine to your strands.

Watch the Shampoo!
Color-treated tresses are especially vulnerable to harsh shampoos. For colors that stick around longer, steer clear of shampooing with anti-dandruff shampoos and strong, sulfate-based shampoo formulas. Opt for gentler formulas that

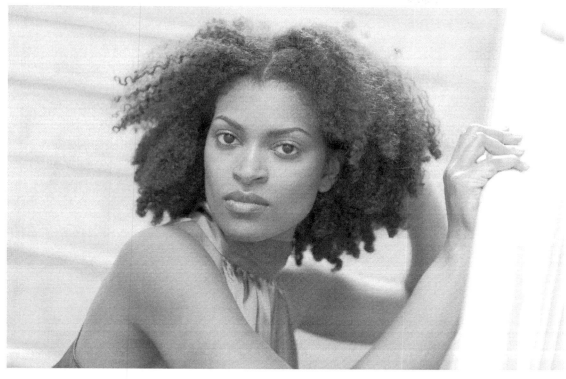

Figure 72- Color-treated hair needs gentle shampoos to keep its color vibrant.

cater to color-treated hair. Volumizing product formulas, while great for thickening up fine strands, can also accelerate the fading process by lifting the cuticle layers ever so slightly to create body.

Cover It!

The sun is a powerful hair bleacher and color lifter. If you're going to be outdoors, protect your color-treated hair with a hat and a touch of sunscreen to shield it from the harsh sun rays. If you're swimming, cover your hair with a swim cap, or saturate it with water and a light conditioner prior to hitting the water. While you won't win any poolside beauty contests, afterward you'll have vibrant color that lasts!

Use Color-Enhancing Products

Spend a few weeks with any new color, and you are bound to lose some vibrancy. Color-enhancing shampoo and conditioner products can buy you and your color a few more weeks of vibrancy! These products work by depositing a small amount of pigment onto the hair during regular washing and conditioning.

Is orangey, brassy hair your problem? Blue/purple shampoos will counteract the red and yellow tones that naturally turn your tresses brassy. You will usually find these shampoos advertised as color brighteners or enhancers for blondes or grays. (Product companies also help us out by putting many of these products in blue or purple packaging and including the words "blue" or "purple" in the products' names (i.e., Aveda *Blue* Malva, Joico Color Endure *Violet* Shampoo)). Just be sure not to abuse these shampoos since they can be drying and will slowly give the hair a bluish undertone!

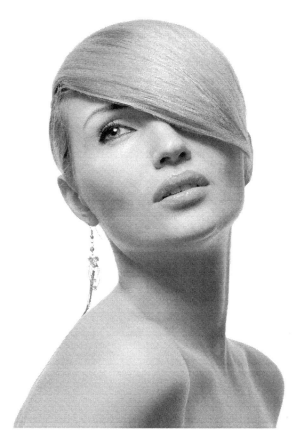

Figure 73- Brassy tones can be fixed with a blue/purple shampoo.

Make It Permanent

While permanent colors have the potential to damage your hair, these colors do remain truer longer. If color longevity is a goal, then a permanent or semipermanent color will hold up to many more shampooings. Permanent pigments reach the cortex and bind with our hair's protein, rather than simply staining the cuticle as rinses and other temporary colors do. Your color-care regimen will need to be solid to accommodate a permanent color, so do proceed with caution.

Avoid Red Tones

Red color pigments are the smallest in size and wash away most easily. While they produce the most vibrant colors right out of the bottle, they fade extra fast!

Contact Dermatitis

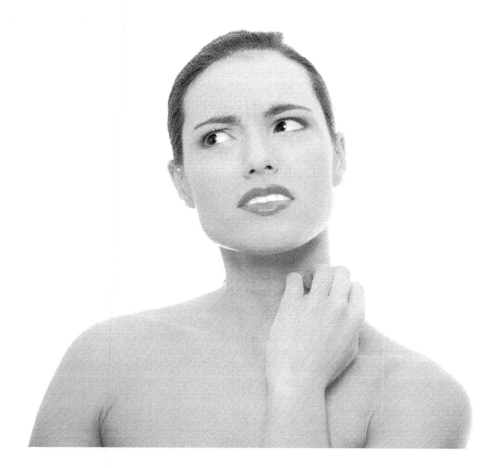

Did your great, new color come with a red, itchy price tag? If you are like 5.7 million Americans, this scenario isn't farfetched or a laughing matter. The lingering, itchy and blistering rashes of contact dermatitis tend to affect females more often than males, and more young adults and teens than any other groups. While contact dermatitis is more commonly associated with problems elsewhere on the skin (the face, neck, ears, and eyelids are the most common sites), the scalp can be affected as well. Fortunately, the tips in this chapter, along with the advice of your medical doctor, can help provide relief for your contact dermatitis.

Signs & Symptoms

Contact dermatitis may appear as slight swelling or warmth in the affected area— or as severe stinging, oozing, crusting, or peeling in affected regions. Common symptoms include

- Swelling, peeling skin.
- Pink or red, itchy skin.
- Dry, flaky skin.

Causes & Triggers

Identifying the exact cause of contact dermatitis is often tricky because a number of irritants may be to blame, and products that were once used without a problem may suddenly become irritants to the body. There are two distinct types of contact dermatitis: *irritant-induced* and *allergen-induced*. Irritant-induced forms of dermatitis respond rather immediately to contact with the problem ingredient, while allergen-induced dermatitis may take one to three days to develop after contact with the problem substance.

Patch testing (similar to a standard allergy test) is generally performed to determine the exact cause of contact dermatitis. Dermatitis triggers vary by region of the body, but for the scalp they generally include:

- Shampoos.
- Hair dyes.
- Topical medications.
- Chemical treatments.
- Irritating fragrances.

Ingredients in hair dyes are the most common instigators of this condition. The chemical ingredient paraphenylenediamine or PPD, found in many permanent hair-dye solutions, is the usual suspect. Cocamidopropyl betaine (commonly found in shampoos) and glyceryl

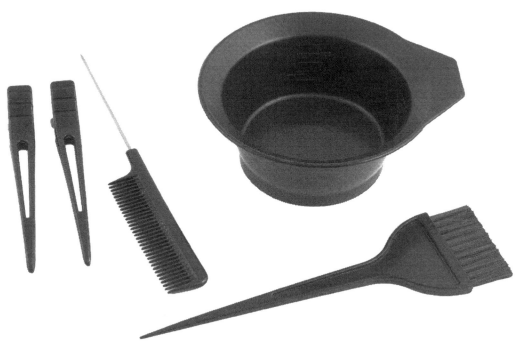

Figure 74- Hair dyes can trigger and aggravate contact dermatitis.

thioglycolate (found in permanent-wave solutions) are also contact-dermatitis triggers. Hairstylists who handle and work with products containing PPD and other irritants often develop contact dermatitis on their hands if they do not wear gloves. With proper treatment and no additional exposure to the irritant, contact dermatitis usually clears up in fourteen to twenty-one days.

When It's Time to See Your Doctor
Check with your doctor if you believe you've developed contact dermatitis. If the condition worsens (rash, swelling, or itchiness spreads to other parts of the body), if there is bleeding, or if there is discomfort, seek medical attention immediately. Although anaphylaxis (a severe allergic reaction that may result in death) is rare, there have been cases of contact dermatitis associated with this condition.

Intervention & Preventing Relapse

Wash Area Immediately

If you have been exposed to a product that you believe has caused contact dermatitis, simply clean the area with soap and cool water to remove the substance and seek medical treatment.

Corticosteroids & Antihistamine Therapy

Corticosteroids are commonly prescribed as creams or ointments to relieve the inflammation from contact dermatitis. If the affected area is particularly large, injectable cortisone or pills may be prescribed instead. Oral antihistamines are also commonly prescribed for contact dermatitis to control itching.

Aloe Vera Therapy

Aloe vera gel is a great, simple remedy for a variety of skin irritations. Apply the gel directly to your irritated skin area 3 to 4 times a day as needed.

Stay Away from Common Irritants

If your skin is suffering from a contact dermatitis flare-up, ensure that your products don't contain these common irritants: PPD, lanolin, cocamidopropyl betaine, glyceryl thioglycolate, neomycin, bacitracin, quaternium-15, para-aminobenzoic acid (PABA), and hydrocortisone cream. Cleanse your hair with gentle, sulfate-free shampoos to avoid further irritation to your sensitive skin.

Conduct a Strand or Patch Test

If you are planning to use chemical treatments, always conduct a strand or patch test prior to use to check for any newly developed allergies. Test yourself even if you've used the product or treatment in question before.

Steer Clear of Fragrances

Although great-smelling products are often desired, synthetic fragrances can also be irritating to those with sensitive skin. Avoiding fragrances in products entirely, however, can be pretty difficult. Almost every commercially available product today contains some kind of fragrance, even those claiming to be unscented! Look for products that are specifically labeled "fragrance-free" for best results.

Cradle Cap

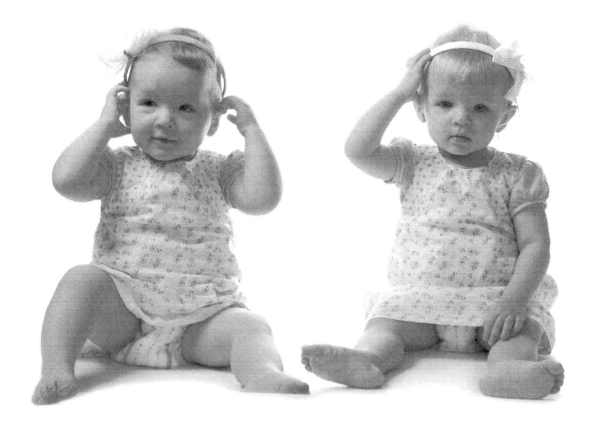

Ten fingers, ten toes, bright, lively eyes . . . and cradle cap? Cradle cap, or seborrheic dermatitis, (in adults) is a painless, temporary skin condition that often looks like thick, scaly, yellowish or brownish skin patches. This condition often affects newborns and toddlers up to age three. Although this flaking, scaly skin condition is not contagious and rarely causes a problem for baby, it can be frustrating for moms and dads. Fortunately, cradle cap tends to clear up in a few months on its own. The tips in this section, used with your pediatrician's approval, may help you relieve cradle cap in your infant.

Signs & Symptoms

- Greasy, yellow or white flakes on the scalp.
- Itchy scalp.
- Scaling made up of hard, greasy flakes that coat the scalp in patches.

Causes & Triggers

For the most part, the cause of cradle cap remains a mystery. Some research has implicated maternal hormones passed on to the baby before delivery as a possible cause of cradle cap. These hormones may cause overproduction of sebum, or oil, on the scalp, which can throw off the scalp skin's balance.

Since many cases of cradle cap respond to antifungal shampoo treatment, many scientists believe that malassezia, the same fungus that instigates regular dandruff, may be to blame for cradle cap in infants.

When It's Time to See Your Doctor
While cradle cap is rarely cute on your baby, it is also rarely bothersome for the child and does not typically require any kind of special medical treatment. Do seek medical attention if the condition worsens—especially if the dry, scaly patches spread to other parts of the body or if there is bleeding associated with the condition.

Intervention & Preventing Relapse

Although cradle cap often clears up on its own, parents (with approval from a pediatrician) can employ a few techniques to move the healing process along.

Loosen the Scales

The scaly skin from cradle cap can be lifted before and after shampooing your baby's hair.

To lift scales before (or without) shampooing: Gently apply baby oil, almond oil, or olive oil to the affected scalp area, and then cover with a warmed, damp towel for about 5 to 10 minutes to soften the scales. If the towel cools before the scales have loosened, carefully rewarm it, testing on yourself first to ensure that it is not too hot for your baby. Some find that leaving the oil alone on the scalp for 15 to 30 minutes gets better scale-lifting results. Rinse out the lifted flakes under water, or dab them out with a soft cloth. If shampooing is not on the schedule, use the damp cloth to try to get off as much of the oil as possible once you've lifted the flakes. Why? Oily scalps tend to hold on to flaking scales. This stickiness can make the scaling and flaking condition worse.

After shampooing the baby's hair: Before rinsing the shampoo from the hair, gently loosen the oily scales with a soft brush, your fingers, or a damp cloth. Rinse off the lifted scales with warm water. Take care not to rub the baby's scalp or pick the scales too vigorously.

Build an Effective Shampoo Regimen

Gently shampoo your baby's scalp several times a week as needed with a mild shampoo formula to help lift and loosen scales that may begin to accumulate on the scalp. Sulfate-free shampoos are best for those who need to shampoo baby's hair and scalp frequently—and they are great for keeping baby's scalp and hair hydrated without encouraging additional dryness. Lightly apply conditioner to baby's hair after each cleansing session. Rinse thoroughly.

Special Shampoos

Stubborn cases of cradle cap may require medicated shampoo. Consult your child's pediatrician for medicated shampoo and treatment suggestions.

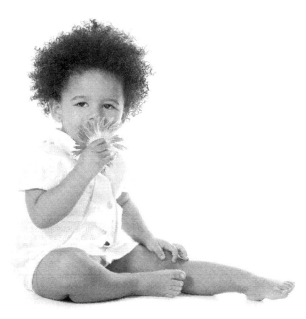

Figure 75- An effective shampoo regimen can reduce the impact of cradle cap.

Daily Massage
Gently massage or brush your little one's head with a soft- bristle brush to improve scalp circulation and to lift dry scales.

Address Biotin Deficiency
Many infants lack certain intestinal flora, or helpful bacteria, in their digestive tracks. These friendly bacteria can help the body absorb biotin, which some evidence has shown may improve cradle cap. Ensuring that nursing mothers receive adequate biotin or B-complex through their diets, or through supplementation, may help resolve cradle cap in their infants.

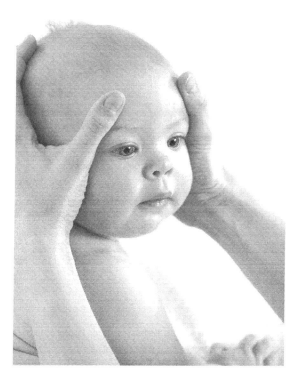

Figure 76- Scalp massage can alleviate cradle cap for your baby.

Crown-Area Hair Breakage

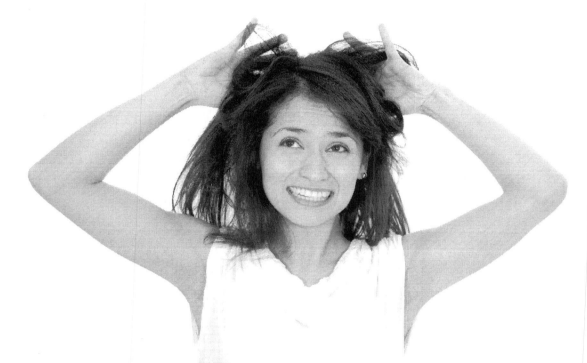

If your hair's hemline is shaped like a W rather than a healthy U or intentional V, you may be suffering from chronic crown-area hair breakage. Crown-area hair breakage, or hair breakage originating from the center of the head, can be very distressing, especially when the rest of the hair is flourishing. Many times, we are simply unaware of the physical trauma that our hair experiences on a daily basis from our styling choices—and often, breakage in areas such as the crown can sneak up on us. The tips in this section may help you resolve your crown-area hair breakage once and for all!

Signs & Symptoms

- Short, broken, uneven hair in the crown area.
- Balding in the crown area.

Causes & Triggers

If your crown-area breakage is not the result of a medical issue, there is hope for restoring the crown's normal fullness and length. The common triggers of crown-area hair breakage are chemical abuse and stressful hairstyling.

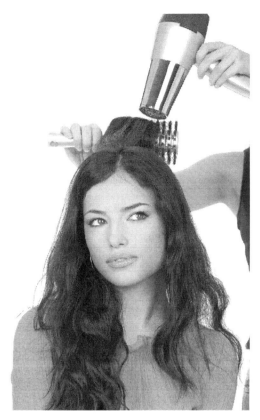

Figure 77- Styling tension in the crown area can lead to breakage.

Chemical abuse includes:

- Overlapping and overprocessing chemical processes such as hair coloring, relaxing, perming or texturizing.

Stressful hairstyling techniques include:

- Using heavy tension when trying to create volume or height at the crown with a round brush.
- Back-combing, teasing, picking out and fluffing the hair with hair tools (combs/ picks).
- Pinning hair in the center/crown repetitively (or putting weight on the crown area with ponytails, hair rollers and buns, etc.).
- Wearing sewn-in weaves, braid extensions and other weaves that have been done too tightly.

- Long-term use of high- pressure shower water.

One other cause of crown-area hair breakage is cicatricial alopecia, or *scarring alopecia*. This is a rare form of alopecia that occurs when the body destroys its own hair follicles and replaces them with scar tissue under the skin's surface. It can occur gradually with no real symptoms over a period of years—or it may cause severe itching and even burning in the crown area. Scarring alopecia eventually leads to permanent hair loss—but catching it in its early stages may prevent it from spreading. Your dermatologist will be able to perform a scalp test to determine if you have the condition.

Intervention & Preventing Relapse
Protein/Moisture Deep Conditioning

Lack of proper conditioning can cause crown-area breakage. Because the top area of the head is exposed to the environment and elements more than any other part, the hair there can really take a beating. The key to restoring hair in the crown area is to isolate the area and pamper it back to life. For restoring crown-area hair, the moisture balance will be your focus. Be sure that you are deep conditioning your hair at least once each week with heat.

When you condition your hair, make sure that you section the hair in small increments so that each and every section of hair, especially the crown, is treated. A surprising number of people simply coat the top and sides of their hair, barely scrunch through the middle of their hair, and slather the ends with conditioner product. For the conditioning to be effective, you have to get in there and make sure the crown area also gets treatment. Similarly, you will want to part through and moisturize the crown area daily with either a protein- or moisture-based moisturizing product.

You really want to focus your conditioning and moisturizing efforts in the middle! It's very easy to miss the crown during moisturizing and conditioning because many of us tend to graze over the top and sides of the hair without really digging in deep to get the underlayers of crown hair. You'd be surprised at the number of people who simply coat the edges, barely scrunch through the middle, and slather the ends with conditioner or moisturizing product. You have to get in there good and make sure the crown area gets some love!

Curl Pattern and Texture Mismatches

It's not uncommon for the crown area to naturally have a slightly different texture or curl pattern from other parts of the head. If your crown area is naturally finer, curlier or coilier than the surrounding strands (or if you are growing out a chemical process), customize your hair care to this fragile area by giving it extra moisturizing and conditioning time.

Massage to Stimulate

To restore blood flow to a sluggish crown, massage your scalp once a day. A nightly ten-minute massage is all you need. You may choose to add stimulating essential oils to your scalp massage for maximum impact. These lightweight oils are great for getting blood flow and nutrients to the scalp and have a calming, relaxing effect as well. Good essential oils to try in your massage are peppermint, lavender, rosemary, and thyme oils. Sweet almond oil and jojoba oil are popular carrier oils that are used to dilute essential oils. Remember, using essential oils in too high a concentration can irritate the scalp.

Beware of Heat

To help restore the crown area and prevent breakage, avoid using direct heat in this area as much as possible. Everyone knows to stay away from blow dryers and flatirons, but when

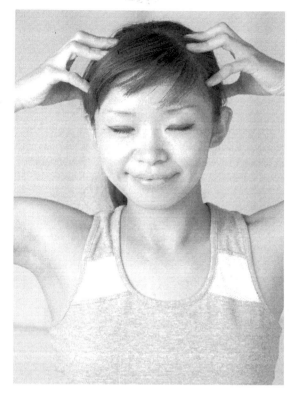

Figure 78- Scalp massage can help bring blood flow back to the crown area.

crown-area breakage is a problem, hooded dryers are often a culprit. Although hooded dryers are considered a safer form of heat, the crown area can still receive a lot of heat attention from a hooded dryer. In fact, the crown area is usually the very first section to dry in most types of wet sets. Make sure that your dryer model circulates heat well and that you are able to adjust the heat settings as needed.

Also allow adequate hair-drying time once your hair is set, so that you can partially air dry your hair. Check your crown regularly as the hair dries. If the crown area dries first, mist it again with water to allow other areas to catch up. Once your hair is about 80 percent dry, come out from under the dryer hood and allow the set to finish drying naturally.

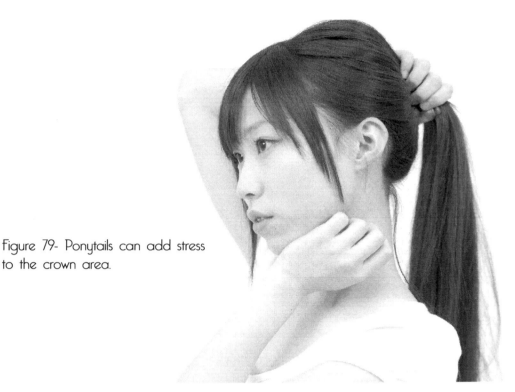

Figure 79- Ponytails can add stress to the crown area.

Chemical Straightening

The crown area is very susceptible to damage from chemical straightening because it sits at the center of the standard four-quadrant sectioning scheme. From the initial application of a relaxer to the rinse out, the crown area is often processed longer than other sections of hair. Reduce your hair's contact with chemicals by stretching out your relaxer applications to no sooner than eight weeks between services. Chemical relaxers should always be applied to the hair carefully—and occasionally, the application sequence should be adjusted to give the crown area a break.

Stressful Hair Styles

Avoid any styles that place tension on the crown area. A slow chronic breakage can occur in the crown area if hair weaves are sewn-in too tightly, rollers are set with too much tension, or the hair is repeatedly rough combed in this area. Ponytails tend to increase crown-area breakage because they often create tension with their placement at the center and back center of the head. When roller setting, place any metal clips needed in the crown area very carefully. Remember that metal clips can get very hot under the dryer and damage the hair.

Straight and free-form styles such as braid-outs (braided hair released as waves), twist-outs (twists released as waves), two-strand twists and roller sets (provided tangling is kept to a minimum) are good for maintaining and growing out a crown.

Discontinuing stressful physical practices will significantly reduce your crown-area breakage.

Damp Hair under Ponytails

Ponytails and buns that are styled on wet or damp hair can weaken the hair over time and may lead to breakage in the middle of the head. If crown-area breakage is a problem for you, try allowing the hair to dry thoroughly before styling the hair in buns or ponytails.

Additional Strategies

To help speed the crown's recovery, here are some additional strategies to consider:

- Cover hair in a satin or silk scarf or bonnet nightly. Avoid cotton bandanas or sleeping on cotton pillows, which can sap precious moisture from your hair.

- Keep the crown area trimmed and as neat on the ends as possible. If your hair is layered, maintaining the evenness of your layers is important. Uneven, splitting, or otherwise frazzled hair easily tangles and can lead to a cycle of intense breakage. Hairs should be able to move freely past other hairs without catching.

Damaged, Highly Porous Hair

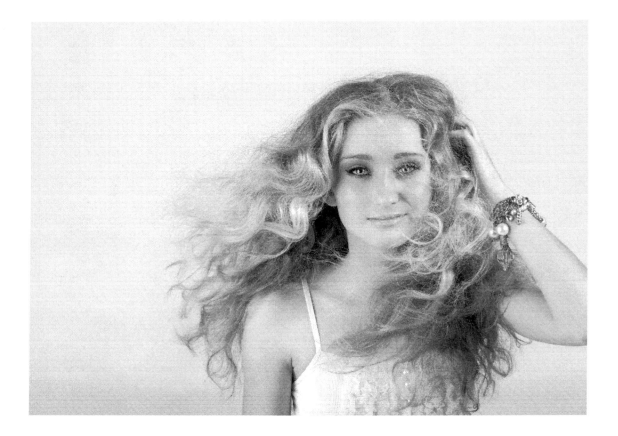

Your hair's ends have seen better days. Travel along the length of your hair, and what starts off as relatively smooth strands near the roots becomes dry, frizzy strands at the tips. It's breaking—and no matter what you do, these strands can't stay moisturized. If things are really bad, your frazzled hair may have already started to become a lighter, brassier or redder shade than your natural hair color. What's worse is that these parched strands are often rebellious and refuse to hold a style. Curl it? *Forget it!* Straighten it? *Not happening!* If this sounds like you, you may have a high-porosity problem. The tips in this section will help you combat damaged, highly porous hair.

Signs & Symptoms

Damaged cuticle layers put up a weak defense against moisture loss, and hair that is frequently parched usually has considerable cuticle-layer damage. Cuticle loss and splitting of the hair fiber contribute to the dull, dry look of porous hair ends. Highly porous hair is:

- Excessively dry.
- Swollen and puffy.
- Dull, lackluster.
- Constantly splitting and breaking.

Too much porosity reduces the hair's ability to hold in moisture, which leaves you with dry, frizzy strands.

Causes & Triggers

The cuticle works very hard to protect the hair's cortex from damage from day-to-day stressors. But the cuticle layers can only take so much trauma before the hair is permanently affected. When the cuticle layers have been stressed to the point of no return, the hair fiber cannot readily respond to protein and moisture conditioning treatments to combat breakage. The more damage your cuticles have endured, the more porous your hair will be. The major causes of increased hair porosity are:

- Heat abuse from styling tools.
- Overprocessing from chemicals.
- Cuticle abrasion from poor-quality combs and brushes.
- Sun overexposure.
- Use of sodium lauryl sulfate or ammonium lauryl sulfate (SLS/ALS)-based shampoos.

The top two causes of high-porosity hair damage are excessive heat use and chemical processing. Heat styling affects the moisture content of the hair and also changes the normal, flat orientation and arrangement of the hair's cuticle layers. Chemical processes must swell the cuticle to deposit pigment or rearrange the hair's protein bonds to achieve curl or straightness. These treatments can cause fracturing, tearing, stripping, and even total cuticle loss.

Intervention & Preventing Relapse

If you can temporarily patch the cuticle damage and constrict the cuticle layers, even a little, you will resolve a majority of your hair porosity issues. Cosmetic fixes are the only real fix for high-porosity problems in hair care. Cuticle scales may be flattened or smoothed again with the help of low-pH conditioners, acidic rinses, and time.

When hair is damaged and porosity is high, both heat use and chemical treatments should be discontinued. Efforts should be concentrated on restoring the hair's internal moisture balance as much as possible, and this first requires diligent protein deep conditioning to rehabilitate the hair's shoddy infrastructure.

Protein Treatments for Porous Hair

The best and perhaps easiest way to patch up damaged cuticle layers is simply through light protein conditioning. Protein fills in gaps, binds to damaged places, and mends individual exterior scales along the cuticle. Regular protein conditioning reduces the hair's porosity by reinforcing the cuticle layers and allowing the hair shaft to better hold on to the moisture it is given.

Acidic Conditioners

Some hair porosity problems can be temporarily resolved by applying a low-pH solution or product—usually a conditioner—to the hair. Most good deep conditioners are acidic products that will help restore and temporarily repair the cuticle layers. After treating the hair with a protein source, your hair should be ready to receive and

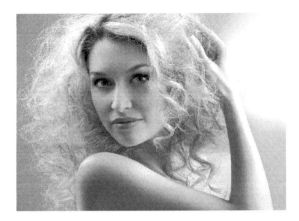

Figure 80- Light protein conditioning can improve dry, porous hair

maintain the moisture you give it from your regular, weekly moisturizing deep conditioner.

When searching for a good acidic shampoo and conditioner brand for your porous hair, check the aisles for products formulated for color-treated hair. Typically, products for color-treated hair are the most acidic and contain small proteins to rebuild the hair shaft. These products are extra gentle and help maintain the tightness of the cuticle layers in order to preserve hair colors and keep vibrant permanent shades from leaching. Even if your hair is not color-treated and you suspect that your hair may be porous, seek out products formulated for damaged or color-treated hair.

Acidic Rinses

A weekly acidic rinse with apple cider vinegar (ACV) is a common home remedy for treating porous hair. Simply combine 1/4 cup apple cider vinegar with 2 cups cool water. Pour this mixture over the hair as a final rinse after shampooing and conditioning are complete. Rinse thoroughly in cool water. This acidic rinse will temporarily reduce porosity by constricting the cuticle scales. The ACV rinse will also enhance your hair's shine, eliminate tangles, and increase manageability. ACV rinses should never make your hair feel hard. If the ACV rinse makes your hair feel hard or tangly after rinsing, your mixture needs to be diluted with more water.

Temporary Color Rinses & Deposit-Only Colors

Temporary clear or colored rinses contain proteins that bind to and patch up the hair shaft. These rinses have the added benefit of enhancing your current hair color or allowing a temporary change. Clear rinses are best if you'd rather keep your current color or just add an enhanced element of shine. Sebastian's Colourshines, Clairol's Jazzings, and body art quality (BAQ) henna are great hair rinses and deposit-only colors that can help reduce your hair's porosity.

Dandruff & Dry Scalp

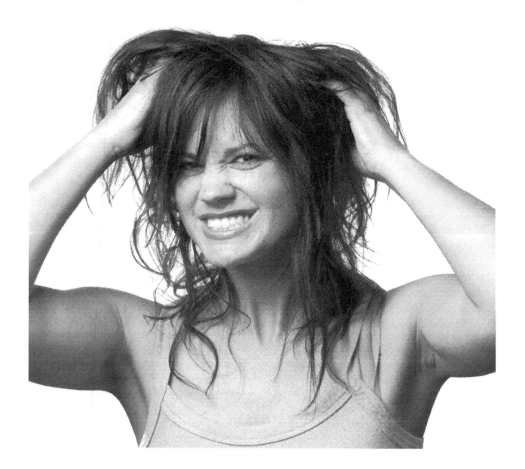

If it seems like you are having a white Christmas each and every day, you are not alone. You may not realize it, but our skin, the scalp included, undergoes a highly organized flaking process on a daily basis. It happens so efficiently that we do not even notice it until something interrupts or slows this shedding process. When skin cells accumulate near the surface of the scalp and are shed at an erratic rate, the result is dandruff. Dandruff is simply excess skin being shed from the scalp. The tips in this section, used with your doctor's approval, may help you relieve your dandruff and dry-scalp issues.

Signs & Symptoms

Dandruff is a pretty straightforward condition to identify. Symptoms commonly include:

- Itchy, flaky skin.
- Dry or oily scalp.

Dandruff and flaking can be categorized as either oily or dry in nature.

Dry dandruff: This type of dandruff flakes easily from the scalp, and the pieces are typically very small.

Oily dandruff: This type of dandruff is the result of the skin cells mixing with the sebum produced by your scalp. This form of dandruff does not flake easily.

Causes & Triggers

Not surprisingly, the causes of dandruff have been debated for years among medical experts. One of the most commonly cited causes of dandruff is the overgrowth of a yeastlike fungus known as *malassezia* on the scalp. Interestingly, *malassezia* also lives on healthy scalps without causing dandruff—but when the fungus grows out of control, dandruff can become a big problem. Scientists are not quite sure why *malassezia* multiplies on the scalp, but many attribute its growth to having excessive amounts of oil on the scalp from infrequent cleansing, having a compromised immune system, or simply experiencing hormonal changes in the body.

Other dandruff causes that have been proposed over the years include:

- Using harsh shampoo products.
- Not fully rinsing conditioners away.
- Eating a poor, high-sugar diet.
- Lack of proper shampooing.

- Inadequate scalp conditioning and hydration.
- Using heavy, oily products on the hair.
- Weather changes (from warm to cold).
- High stress.

When It's Time to See Your Doctor
Most dandruff cases do not need to be treated by a doctor. However, if weeks of treatment with antidandruff shampoos still leave you with pesky flakes, or if you notice swelling or redness along the scalp or neck, it may be time to schedule a visit with your doctor or dermatologist. Your dandruff may only be a symptom of a larger scalp problem.

Is It Just Dandruff?

Several scalp conditions have been known to mimic dandruff or to have dandruff as a primary symptom.

Psoriasis

Scalps with psoriasis tend to have thick, silvery, scaly skin. Although other parts of the body can be affected by psoriasis, the scalp is the most frequently affected region of the skin. While psoriasis of the scalp also often leads to some hair loss, many sufferers never have any symptoms other than scalp scaling.

Seborrheic Dermatitis

Nearly 30 percent of Americans suffer from seborrheic dermatitis, but they often are not aware of it. This condition mimics dandruff so closely that many sufferers commonly mistake it for a really bad case of dandruff. Seborrheic dermatitis is characterized by a dry, itchy scalp with thick, flaky patches of skin forming primarily around the perimeter of the scalp. These scaly flakes may even form around and attach to the base of the hair shaft. Cradle cap (see page 128) is a form of seborrheic dermatitis that develops in infancy. This condition tends to run in families.

Intervention & Preventing Relapse

Dandruff can be controlled in most cases, but patience and persistence will be required to continue seeing long-term results.

Treat Dandruff from the Inside

Diet plays a role in the frequency of dandruff flare-ups. If your diet lacks zinc, vitamin A, B vitamins, or certain types of fats, dandruff is more likely to affect you. Increasing the percentage of raw foods (fresh vegetables and fruits) you consume has been found to alleviate dandruff in some individuals.

For the dry type of dandruff, supplementing your diet with a tablespoon of flaxseed oil every morning may help turn around your dandruff trouble. Flaxseed oil is also a proven remedy for dry skin. If your dandruff is of the oily variety and readily sticks to your scalp in patches, skip the flaxseed-oil remedy.

Special Shampoos

Zinc pyrithione, ketoconazole, and selenium sulfide shampoos are anti-dandruff formulas that are designed to quickly lift and remove flaking scales from both dry and oily dandruff types.

If these types of shampoo do little for your dandruff, consider upgrading to a tar-based shampoo. Used as a dandruff remedy for well over two centuries, tar shampoos have been found to decrease skin cell turnover and flaking. A prescription-strength tar shampoo may be needed for stubborn and oily forms of dandruff. Small flare-ups may be cleared up with a mild over-the-counter tar shampoo formula.

Use your specially formulated dandruff shampoo once and follow it up with a 30-minute deep conditioning. Repeat in three to four days with a gentle (non-dandruff) shampoo, and deep condition the hair again. To prevent resistance to your medicated shampoo, consider alternating different shampoos with different

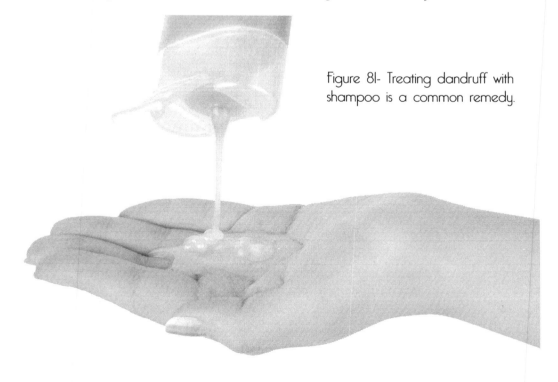

Figure 81- Treating dandruff with shampoo is a common remedy.

active ingredients each month. (For example, in Month 1, use a zinc pyrithione–based shampoo. In Month 2, use a selenium sulfide–based shampoo, etc.)

Examples of Various Dandruff Shampoos

- **Zinc pyrithione shampoos**
  Head & Shoulders

- **Tar-based shampoos**
  Neutrogena T/Gel

- **Selenium sulfide shampoos**
  Selsun Blue

- **Ketoconazole shampoos**
  Nizoral

Deep Conditioning

Applying heavy oils and pomades to the hair and scalp is a common practice for fixing dry scalp issues and provides temporary relief—but this practice often only encourages the cycle of dandruff and dryness to continue. Dandruff should be controlled by hydrating the scalp with water, not by merely lubricating it with oil.

Gentle cleansing and deep conditioning can alleviate dandruff flare-ups. While deep conditioning works wonders for the hair, deep-conditioning treatments also benefit the scalp with the moisture they provide. When we use harsh shampoos, especially those with sulfate-based cleansers, these products can leave our scalps feeling dry and tight. Be sure to deep condition your hair at least once per week with a moisturizing deep conditioner to maintain the moisture balance in your scalp and hair.

Dandruff-Fighting Vinegar Rinses

Vinegar rinsing is a natural remedy that has been found to cure dandruff in some individuals.

To relieve dandruff and help restore the scalp's natural pH balance, try a vinegar rinse after your shampoo.

In a bottle combine ½ cup apple cider vinegar, ½ cup aloe vera gel, and 2 cups spring water. Apply to the hair and scalp, and massage gently. Allow the mixture to sit on the scalp for 3 minutes, and then rinse well with warm water. Follow the treatment with your favorite conditioner.

Vinegar Rinsing (after Conditioner)

You may also use the vinegar rinse described above as a final rinse after you have conditioned your hair.

Massage

Massage naturally encourages increased blood flow and circulation to sluggish areas of the scalp. Scalp massages are especially effective when combined with stimulating essential oils to combat dandruff. Avoid scratching the scalp as you massage. Some forms of excessive dandruff such as psoriasis are aggravated by the trauma caused by itching.

Essential Oils

NOTE: Always consult a physician prior to trying essential oils, especially if you are a woman who is pregnant or nursing.

Great essential oils for massaging away your dandruff problems are tea tree, lavender, lemongrass, neem and rosemary. You may use one or a combination of these oils for your dandruff treatment. Essential oils should be used only in increments of 3 to 4 drops at a time and must be diluted in a thicker oil prior to use on the scalp skin. This thicker oil is known as a "carrier" oil because it carries the essential oil and helps to spread it out over a larger coverage area. Sweet almond oil, olive oil, jojoba oil and melted coconut oil work well as carrier oils in most mixtures.

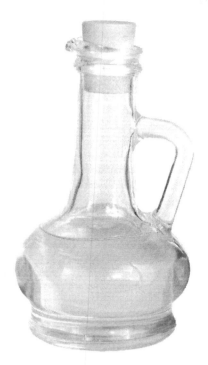

Figure 82- Vinegar rinsing is a natural remedy for dandruff.

Proper dilution is the key. Generally, you need just enough carrier oil to prevent burning or irritation from the strong essential oil. Slowly add I drop of the essential oil at a time to the carrier oil, testing between drops to insure that the proper dilution for your personal tolerance level is met. Adding 2 to 3 drops of essential oil diluted in about 2 tablespoons carrier oil is a great starting mixture. You can easily adjust the mixture to your taste. Warming your carrier oil beforehand will enhance your essential oil experience.

Tea tree oil is by far the most popular natural remedy for dandruff. For a simple mixture, add 2 tablespoons of tea tree oil to ½ cup or more of jojoba or olive oil. Any carrier oil can be used to suit your preference.

Using the essential oil mixture just prior to cleansing with a regular shampoo is one of the best ways to combat dandruff. Apply your essential oil mixture to your scalp and massage for 10 to 20 minutes. Allow the oils to penetrate your scalp for 5 additional minutes, and then shampoo with a medicated, anti-dandruff shampoo. Condition your hair as normal, taking great care to ensure you have rinsed the hair and scalp thoroughly.

Gingerroot Scalp Spritzer

To fight dandruff, finely grate half a gingerroot into 2 cups of water and boil until it is reduced to I cup of tea. Add in I tablespoon *each* lemon juice and olive oil. Mist the scalp and let dry before shampooing it out. You may also use the gingerroot spritzer as

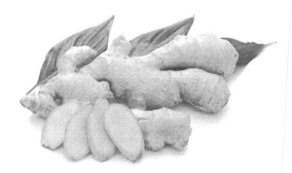

Figure 83- Ginger is a natural scalp soother.

an overnight treatment 2 to 3 times per week to alleviate dandruff problems.

Dry, Brittle Hair

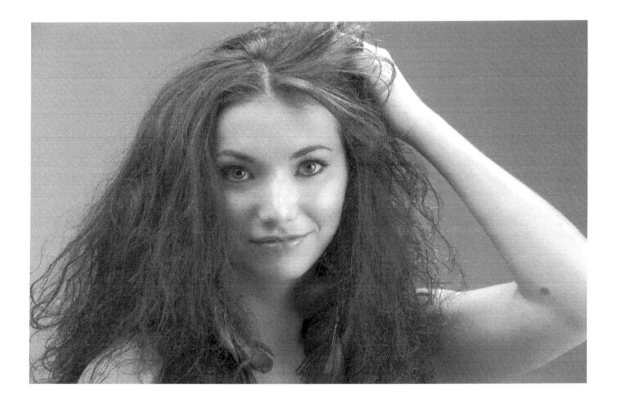

Does it feel like you are wearing a permanent straw hat? Dry, crunchy, brittle hair is a common hair complaint for people the world over. Many times, dry, brittle hair is simply hair that has been overworked, dehydrated, or improperly sealed to retain hydration. Other times, dry hair is a symptom of a larger health issue. Our bodies produce a line of defense against dry, brittle hair—sebum. Unfortunately for many of us, this precious, lipid-rich oil typically never makes it to the ends of our hair for a variety of reasons. If your hair looks and feels like the Sahara Desert at the end of the day, you are not alone. The tips in this section will help you say goodbye to dry, crunchy, brittle hair and hello to hydration once and for all!

Signs & Symptoms

- Excessive hair dryness.
- Swollen, puffy hair.
- Dull, lackluster hair.
- Rampant hair breakage.

Causes & Triggers

Dry, brittle hair is usually a direct result of overworking or overstyling the hair so that the cuticle loses its ability to prevent moisture loss. Contrary to popular belief, oils (including sebum) are not the moisture our hair needs. Oils simply help to keep the moisture our hair naturally contains, secured within the fiber. Any change to

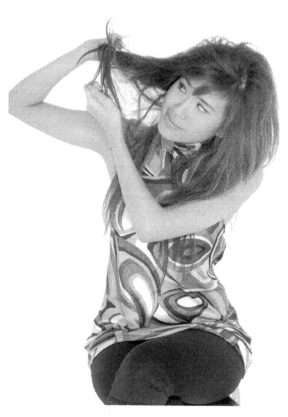

Figure 84- Overworking the hair can result in dryness and brittleness.

the cuticle or its protective oil barrier will result in dryness. The top causes of hair dryness are:

- Excessive physical and chemical abuse.
- The natural shape of the hair fiber.
- Improper product usage.
- Certain health conditions and diet.
- Environmental factors.

Physical and Chemical Abuse

Physical and chemical abuse from excessive heat styling, brushing, perming, relaxing and coloring damages the hair by seriously frazzling and breaking down the hair's protective outer layer. When the hair's outer layer is fried, the hair's porosity increases. Dry, brittle hair is almost always highly porous hair, which means that the hair absorbs and then releases moisture unopposed. The hair fibers can't hold onto their moisture, and so moisture is always being lost from the strands to the environment. Not only do frazzled cuticles have a harder time keeping moisture in the hair, they also have a harder time reflecting light back to the eyes than smooth, flattened cuticles. This poor light reflection makes hair appear even drier.

Hair Fiber Shape

Sometimes the natural shape of our hair fibers can lead to dryness or at least, *to the look of dryness*. Waves, curls, and coils tend to have slightly lifted cuticles at the strands' bending points, which can lead to higher porosity and drier-feeling hair. Often these hair types also have the most trouble getting natural oils from the scalp down through to the ends because of the complex curling and coiling of the hair fibers. In chemically straightened coily hair, new growth can stop sebum distribution right in its tracks! Finally, curlier hair types can also look drier because light does not reflect as intensely from the surface as it does with straighter hair.

Improper Product Use

Our products can either help us or hurt us when we are trying to repair dry, brittle hair. When dry hair is caused by improper product use, a number of factors can contribute to the condition:

- Stripping shampoo products—especially sodium lauryl sulfate or ammonium lauryl sulfate shampoos.
- Mineral oil and petrolatum in moisturizing and finishing products.

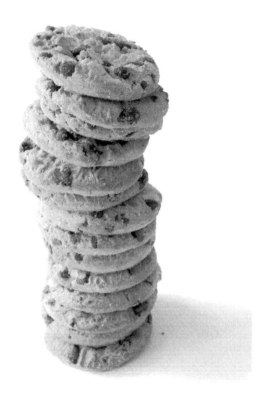

figure 85- Poor diet choices can lead to dry, brittle hair

- Low-impact conditioners.
- Products that are not pH balanced (i.e., products under pH 3.5 or over pH 6).
- Alcohol-based finishing or sculpting products.
- Protein-based reconstructing products.
- Humectant-rich hair products, especially in arid climates.

Health Conditions

Certain health conditions may also lead to dry, brittle hair in some individuals. When these conditions are treated or managed, hair dryness will improve. These health issues include

- Underactive thyroid (hypothyroidism).
- Eating disorders such as anorexia or bulimia.
- Poor nutrition.
- Crash dieting/restrictive food group dieting.

Hypothyroidism is a common health-related cause of dry, brittle hair. (Brittle nails, weight gain, fatigue and feeling cold are other common symptoms of this condition.) In addition to eating disorders that can completely disrupt the flow of nutrients to the body, a simple lack of protein in the diet can result in dry, brittle hair. Iron, biotin, Vitamin A and Vitamin C deficiencies can also lead to naturally parched strands as the hair grows in.

Environmental Factors

It doesn't take a rocket scientist to see that climate plays a role in how our hair feels. Dry, arid climates—hot or cold can cause hair to feel parched and dry. Sun exposure and exposure to cold, crisp air can lead to dryness in all hair types. Hard water is also a common environmental culprit that can lead to dry, coated-feeling hair.

> **When It's Time to See Your Doctor**
> If your hair dryness is accompanied by hair loss or is paired with additional symptoms, you should consult a physician.

Intervention & Preventing Relapse

Go Easy on the Chemicals

There's no faster way to get a new look than coloring, perming or relaxing the hair—but these are also surefire ways to damage and dry it out as well. If you must chemically process the hair for your new look, be sure to only work with hair that is in tip-top condition. Processing damaged hair can lead to even more trouble than it's worth—plus, services always look better on healthy hair. Avoid double-processing (treating with more than one chemical at a time, i.e., coloring plus perming) whenever possible because this increases hair porosity and, of course, dryness significantly.

Say No to Heat

Thermal hair treatments are all the rage these days, but using heat on your hair is the world's fastest way to dry it out. If you suffer from problems with dry hair, cut out the daily heat and opt for a safer form of drying with a blow dryer diffuser attachment, hooded dryer or, even better, air drying. If you will be using heat, always use a heat protectant first on well-conditioned hair.

Evaluate Your Shampoo

Shampoos are the number-one product culprit for dry hair. Shampoos, especially those that are sulfate-based, are excellent cleansers and can lift varying degrees of hair product from the hair. Unfortunately, along with this amazing product lift comes the near-complete removal of the hair's natural lubricant: sebum. Without sebum, the hair is unprotected, hair fibers cannot move easily past one another, and the entire hair shaft appears dull.

While regular shampooing-and-conditioning sessions are a good thing, each wash swells the hair and removes precious oils. Be sure that you are replacing lost oils and lipids by following all washing sessions with a conditioner as needed.

Go on a Moisture-Seeking Mission

Lay out your hair care products and start reading product labels! Any products that you find with sulfates, SD alcohols, petrolatum, mineral oil, or heavy oils and silicones such as castor oil and dimethicone need to go! These product ingredients are key moisture robbers. Sulfates strip precious oils from our hair, and mineral oil and similar lubricating ingredients quickly create thick layers on the hair that prevent it from receiving vital moisture. In general, moisturizers for hair should contain water and a few humectants and emollients for moisture support before you ever get to oils or silicones in the list. Common humectants and emollients include aloe vera, glycerin, and ceramides.

Invest in a Heavy-Duty Deep Conditioner

Hair needs to be nourished and surrounded in gentle, light, cuticle-smoothing emollients. For those with dry, brittle hair, lifted and missing cuticle scales are a key problem. To turn around dry hair, moisture must be pumped into the fiber, and then cuticle repair and smoothing must follow. Deep condition your hair with a moisturizing deep conditioner mixed with a small amount of a light protein conditioner. Condition the hair with heat for 10 to 15 minutes, and then rinse in cool water.

Test Your Water & Get pH under Control

Hard water is often a hidden cause of severely dry hair. The dissolved minerals (usually calcium and magnesium) in hard water can bind to our hair and dry it out considerably. Consider investing in a water softener or filtration system to remove the harsh minerals/metals. Water-hardness testing can be conducted free of charge. As of this writing, www.budgetwater.com offers free water testing; simply mail in your water sample.

Also, test the pH of your commonly used products to ensure that they are within the

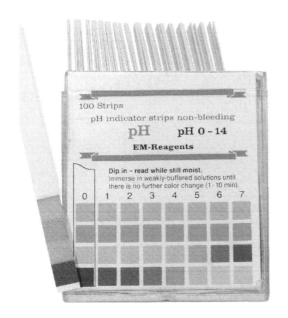

Figure 86- High-pH hair products can lead to dry, brittle hair.

healthy 3.5 to 6 pH range. You can usually find pH test strips at your local drug store. Our hair's pH is naturally in the acidic 4.0 to 5.5 range, so products formulated within this range will keep it healthy.

Weather Watch!

Unfortunately, dry, brittle hair can affect us in both the warmer and the cooler months! Harsh summer rays can sap precious moisture from our stands, and crisp, cold winter air can also ravage our tresses. When weather is extreme, consider protecting the hair with a light, fashionable scarf or hat. Interestingly, products that contain humectants (the product ingredients that normally draw moisture to the hair) can also lead to dryness in different types of weather. When the dew point is fairly low (40°F range and below), humectants like glycerin pull moisture from the hair into the air, which can lead to dryness. To combat this, simply avoid using moisturizers in which glycerin is one of the top-three items in the ingredients list—or ensure that your glycerin-and-water mixtures are heavy on the water during the colder months.

Mask It!

Avocados are a great way to infuse your tresses with natural moisture. Try the Avocado Hair Mask recipe from the Special Hair Conditioning & Restoration Treatments section of this book.

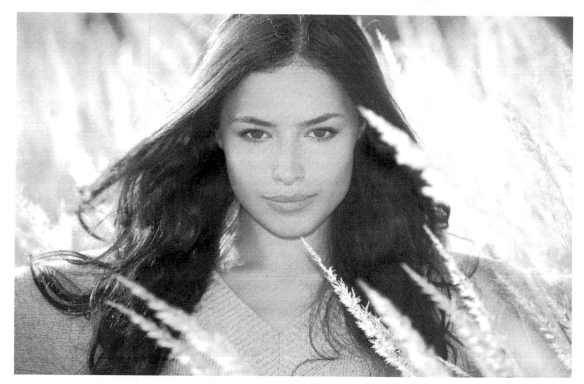

Figure 87- Weather conditions are prime contributors to dry, brittle hair.

Eczema & Red, Itchy Scalp

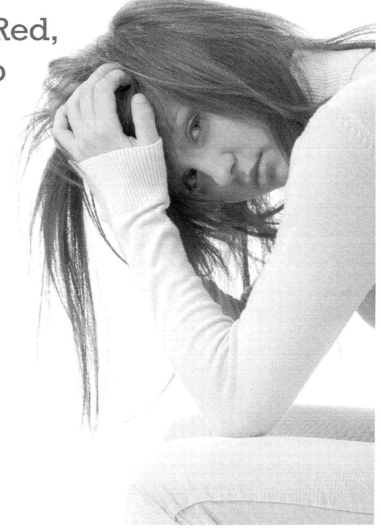

sk anyone with eczema, and they will tell you it's no walk in the park. Eczema flare-ups usually result in excessively itchy, dry, red skin that may blister, burn, or form thick, scaly crusts. Eczema is a noncontagious form of dermatitis that is brought on by allergic reactions to pollen, food, dry air, and many other things. Although eczema can occur on any part of the body, the scalp is one of the more commonly affected areas. Fortunately, the tips in this section, used with your doctor's approval, may help you relieve your eczema and red, itchy scalp issues.

Signs & Symptoms

Although eczema can affect people of any gender and age, it is most common in girls and children under five. Since it is a chronic condition, eczema can reappear in later life in those who were affected as children. What's worse is that the condition can often spring up without notice. Common signs and symptoms of eczema include:

- Tender, itchy scalp.
- Red, blistered skin.
- Dry, scaly crusts.

Causes & Triggers

The exact cause of eczema is not well known, but a number of theories exist. Some researchers believe that an impaired immune system, combined with a possible genetic defect in skin, is responsible for eczema outbreaks. Allergies to certain fragrances, detergents, soaps, clothing, and even sweat have been found to trigger some types of eczema. High emotional stress and changes in temperature have also been cited as the cause of some eczema outbreaks.

When It's Time to See Your Doctor
If your scalp condition persists or becomes worse, it may be time to see your doctor. Seek medical attention immediately if you develop signs of infection such as extreme redness, swelling, soreness, or fever, or if long-term treatment options are ineffective.

Intervention & Preventing Relapse
Cleanse the Hair with Care
Regular cleansing is vital to maintaining our hair. However, too frequent shampooing and conditioning may actually aggravate skin with eczema if proper precautions are not taken.

Take care to avoid scratching the scalp during cleansing as this may lead to further irritation. Shampoos should always be sulfate-free, and long conditioning sessions (>15 minutes) should be avoided to prevent overexposure to water. Using steam to deep condition the hair (via hooded steaming devices) may also aggravate the skin and trigger problems in some people who battle with eczema outbreaks. Any conditioners applied to the hair should be rich in *ceramides* or *lipids* to help reinforce the uppermost layer of skin.

Moisturize & Seal
With healthy scalp skin, it is not advisable to place heavy oils directly on the scalp as this can hamper its normal functioning. However, with eczema, the uppermost layer of skin is unable to fulfill its usual barrier function and cannot prevent moisture loss on its own. When this skin is treated with moisture, the rapid evaporation of this moisture back into the environment can lead to flare-ups of the condition. Barrier products such as oil-based moisturizers and natural oils placed directly on the scalp help to support the skin and keep moisture inside.

Daily water-based moisturizing of the scalp and hair with combination moisturizing products containing both water and oil is a great way to manage scalp skin that is prone to eczema outbreaks. After cleansing and conditioning the scalp, any eczema treatment prescribed by your doctor should be applied to the affected area, and then a light moisturizer or oil should be applied immediately thereafter to seal the skin. Prescription medication and doctor-prescribed treatments must always be applied to the skin before any other commercial hair products and preparations. For moisture on non-wash days, gently mist the affected scalp areas with water and follow the moisture in one to three minutes

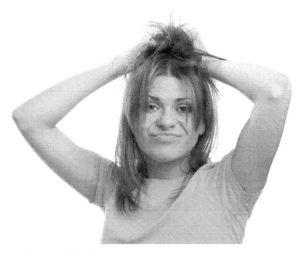

Figure 88- The cause of eczema is still not well known.

with a barrier moisturizing cream or oil product such as coconut, olive or jojoba oil.

Avoid Mineral Oil & Lanolin

Although many hair care products are chock full of mineral oil and lanolin, these ingredients are common eczema irritants. To keep flare-ups to a minimum, avoid mineral oil and lanolin in your hair products. Instead, opt for hair- and scalp-friendly oils such as coconut, olive or jojoba and similar butter products.

Control Eczema with Diet

Some eczema cases can be controlled with diet. (Interestingly, some of the foods commonly associated with instigating outbreaks in some sufferers also play a role in keeping the condition at bay for non-allergic sufferers of eczema.) Dairy products, nuts, seafood, and wheat products have all been found to encourage eczema outbreaks in some sufferers. Eliminate foods that you think may be contributing to outbreaks one at a time for a week or two. Strategic elimination of potential food offenders will help you pinpoint the likely food culprits that trigger your eczema outbreaks. Once you determine the food or foods that bring on symptoms, avoid them to keep breakouts few and far between.

Try a Little Sun Therapy

Some cases of eczema benefit from brief, controlled bouts of sun exposure. Direct sun therapy (or heliotherapy) works best for eczema sufferers when it is combined with other treatments and if it is done many times each day for short exposure times of 5 to 10 minutes or less. Always protect exposed areas of skin that are not affected by eczema with sunscreen, and avoid extended periods in the sun. Hair styles such as cornrows or braids with multiple partings in the hair naturally lend themselves to direct sun therapy, but for those with other hairstyles and those who prefer to avoid direct sun exposure, artificial sunlight via phototherapy may be a better option.

Hand-held phototherapy wands, combs, and brushes have shown some success in alleviating eczema symptoms in studies. Hand-held treatment reduces the risks that direct sun exposure entails, allows for longer periods of treatment if desired, and also allows for treatment in less sunny climates. These treatments can be done at home or in a doctor's office.

Check with your doctor to determine if you are a good candidate for light therapy. Sun and phototherapy may not be a good option for you if

- You are pregnant.
- You have lupus or any other condition that gets worse with light exposure.
- You are at an increased risk for skin cancer.
- You are taking medications that make the skin more sensitive to light (oral contraceptives, high blood pressure medications, and some antibiotics).

Hand-held phototherapy machines can be purchased for home use for $30 to $100, but some units, depending on the brand, can go as high as several thousand dollars. Paying more for your equipment may not guarantee a better product—so check with your doctor for brand recommendations. Also, be sure to check with your insurance provider as some of your equipment costs may be covered by your insurance.

Fish Oil Therapy

The experts continue to debate whether or not fish oil is truly beneficial to eczema sufferers, but some research has shown that the oil does have protective effects for some people. Fish oil taken as a supplement provides relief by reducing the skin's inflammatory response.

Fish oil comes in a variety of forms including

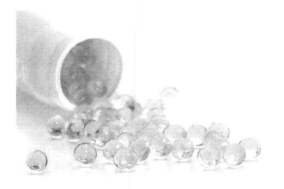

Figure 89- Fish oil has been touted by some as an eczema reliever.

capsules, liquid, and even a chewable variety. Flaxseed oil, hemp seed oil, and evening primrose oil (available at your local health food store) are alternatives to fish oil that contain the beneficial Omega-3 fatty acids that fish oil provides. Always consult with your doctor prior to taking any new supplements, especially if you take blood-thinning medications. A doctor or nutritionist can recommend dosing that is suitable for your situation. Taking too much fish oil can increase levels of vitamin A in the body, and there's an increased danger of toxicity if supplements are not taken in the proper proportion.

Yogurt Therapy

While dairy products instigate eczema in some sufferers, emerging research has shown that active ingredients, known as *probiotics*, in some yogurt

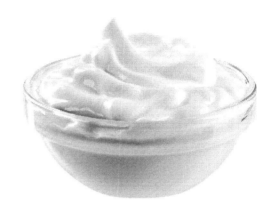

Figure 90- Some types of yogurt may be effective at alleviating eczema symptoms in some sufferers.

brands may help reduce the incidence and severity of eczema in other sufferers. In particular, the probiotic *Lactobacillus rhamnosus* found in some yogurt varieties has shown promise as an eczema reliever in young children. A serving a day of yogurt will suffice to reap the benefits of this treatment.

Sulfur Therapy

Sulfur is another natural treatment that has been found to relieve symptoms of eczema with some success. The body's own natural supply of sulfur supports collagen production, which is essential for maintaining skin elasticity. Eating a diet high in natural sources of sulfur including eggs, lean meat, soybeans, garlic, onions, fish, cabbage, cheese, and poultry—provided, of course, that none of the foods listed above are your personal eczema triggers—may be beneficial for relieving eczema flare-ups.

Fine, Limp Hair

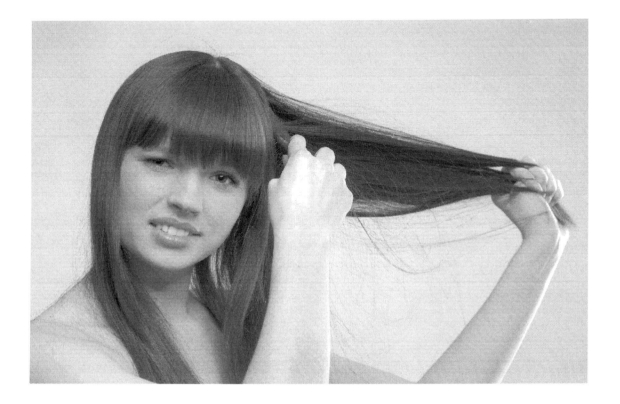

Y ou may have inherited your mother's beautiful eyes and your father's charming wit and smile—but who asked for Aunt Mabel's limp, lank hair? Seriously, it is the pits! Limp hair is simply hair that lacks body and movement, either due to genetics or improper product selection. Naturally fine hair also tends to be naturally oily, limp hair. Fine hairs are small, so it takes many, many more of them to cover the same area of scalp as thicker strands. Since each hair comes equipped with its own oil-producing gland machine, more hairs equal more oil glands! While there won't be much you can do to undo the limp hair you inherited from your family, the tips in this section may help you add new life to your limp strands!

Signs & Symptoms

Fine, limp hair usually has a difficult time holding a style on its own. When it's allowed to grow long, it tends to hang lifelessly unless efforts are taken to volumize it! These are common signs and symptoms of fine, limp hair:

- Hair falls flat.
- Small diameter hair strands, but lots of them.
- Usually straight.
- Often oily, but not always.
- Usually blonde.

Causes & Triggers

Fine, limp hair tends to be passed down the family line or is encouraged by the use of products that linger on the hair strands and weigh them down. Blondes tend to have the finest hair strands of all. The major causes of limp hair are:

- Genetics, natural hair trait.
- Overuse of products such as oils and serums.
- Using a conditioner product that is too heavy, or too rich in oils, for your hair type.
- Hard water.
- Improper selection of finishing products.

Intervention & Preventing Relapse
Cut & Style

The proper haircut and shape can make all the difference for flat, limp tresses. Hair that is all one length will always make hair look flat. Add height and dimension to your hair with a layered cut. Layered cuts will allow your hair to move better and give the appearance of additional fullness. Layers work very well for all hair lengths.

Roller sets are also a great style for building volume into limp, lank hair.

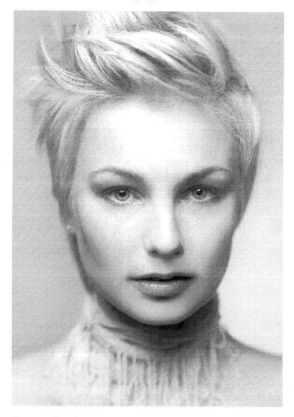

Figure 91- A great cut can improve the look of fine. limp hair.

Although coloring can be damaging to fine hair, if the hair is well cared for, coloring can actually be beneficial for plumping up fine, limp hair in some cases. Coloring—particularly going lighter—has the bonus benefit of slightly swelling the hair, so it appears thicker and has more texture. If the color is done strategically—with highlighting, for example—this can also give the appearance of fuller hair. With proper care, this added texture and dimensional color can give a little boost to desperately limp strands.

Pump up the Volume

Limp hair needs a careful balance of both volumizing and moisturizing products to look its best. If your hair is naturally fine or has a tendency to hang lifelessly, look for lightweight volumizing shampoo and conditioner formulas

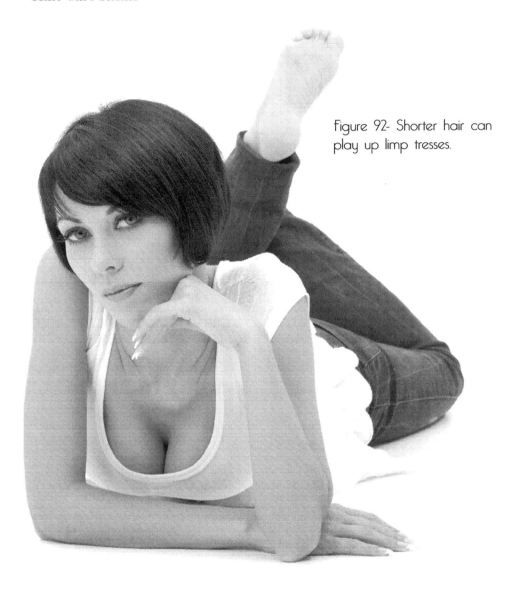

Figure 92- Shorter hair can play up limp tresses.

to add texture and thickness to your hair. If you've decided to color away your limpness, one downside that you've probably noticed is that some volumizing product brands can work against color retention and quickly fade your hair color. On the flip side, many color-treated shampoo and conditioner formulas are simply too heavy for fine or oily hair. Unfortunately, this can leave many color-treated folks with fine hair choosing between getting a volume boost and keeping their color vibrant.

Chelate & Clarify Your Hair

Hair that begins to feel limp and lank may be suffering from hard water build up. If you live in a hard water area, chelating your hair every month or so (see Chapter 5 for more on this) will help to remove dulling hard water deposits that build up on your hair from your shower water. Hair that is naturally fine also easily falls victim to this kind of buildup! If the problem with your water is really bad, consider purchasing a shower filter or using rain or spring water to cleanse your hair.

If you think your buildup issue is product related, clarifying the hair will lift stubborn product residues that can weigh down our hair, making it look limp and lank. Oils, custards, serums, pomades, and silicone-based products are known for building up on the hair fiber and should be removed by clarifying once or twice per month. If the hair is excessively oily, a quick rinsing with water (or full cleansing with a daily shampoo) several times per week can eliminate some of the weight caused by natural hair oils.

Reverse Condition the Hair

Fine hair does benefit from conditioning when it's done the right way! Keeping your fine hair properly conditioned will also control flyaways and add shine. Focus your conditioning products along the middle-length and ends of the hair (basically your ponytail area) to keep a little lift at the roots and base of the hair. Always rinse out conditioners extremely well.

If most conditioners still leave you flat and lifeless, consider reverse conditioning your hair—that is, applying your conditioner first and then lightly shampooing it out of your hair. This way, you can leave in as much (or as little) conditioning agent as you need to avoid the unwanted flatness, but still prevent flyaways and static issues from lack of conditioning. If your hair detangles easily after rinsing your shampoo, you may be able to skip the traditional conditioning step altogether.

Avoid Overloading Your Hair

Hair that is fine-textured or has a tendency toward limpness is also easily weighed down with after-shampoo products. Go light on your styling products! It is always best to use too little product than too much when adding finishing touches to the hair. You can always add a little more product later if needed. Styling creams and lotions that contain heavy conditioning and shaft-coating ingredients (like silicones) can weigh fine hair down, making your hair look flat. Add more body and volume to your tresses after shampooing by using a foam or spray specifically formulated to add volume to the hair.

If you like to use finishing sprays to lock in your style—for light, touchable hold, simply spray a bit of your product into the air and walk into the mist you've created. This works great with most aerosol sprays (as well as perfume!)

TIP: Whenever possible, look for alcohol-free volume products. Alcohol-free products will give you lift without dryness. The downside is that they may take a bit longer to dry on the hair.

Start in the Back

How do most people apply their hair products? Well, most of us are *slatherers*. We slather hair products onto the tops of our heads first, then distribute throughout the hair. But if your hair is fine or limp, this slathering method will only make matters worse for you! To preserve as much volume as possible, you'll want to start product application with much less product and always at the back of your head first. Distribute the product in your hands first to avoid overusing products in your hair, work your way around the sides, and then finally to the top.

Blow in Your Lift

Although blow dryers, when used in excess, can be hard on all hair types—they are still excellent volume boosters. When you blow dry your hair, bend your head down and blow underneath your hair to get incredible lift at the roots. Use a good vented brush to help air circulate and direct the air to create more lift. Lightly blow hair against the direction it will be falling in your finished style, and be sure to gently lift the hair out and away from the head while you are drying. Enhance the lift by applying a pump or two of volume mousse to your damp roots beforehand.

Once dry, flip your head back and finish your style with a light misting of hairspray—again, walk into the mist!

Play around with Partings

One quick way to add a bit of volume to flat hair is to change how you part your hair. If you are used to a center part, try a side or diagonal part to build more volume at the base of your hair and to add some lift at the crown.

Dietary Considerations

If your hair is limp, it may be time to revamp your dietary situation. Undernourished follicles produce undernourished hair. If you are lacking certain vitamins and minerals, taking a basic one-a-day vitamin can get you on the proper footing so that you produce thicker, sturdier hair shafts.

Chemically-Relaxed Hair?

Try the Mid-Relaxer Protein Step. The chemical-relaxing process is well known for its ability to seriously flatten textured hair and make it limp. For those who relax their hair, the mid-relaxer protein step works well for quickly restoring weight and movement to freshly relaxed tresses. After thoroughly rinsing your relaxer, apply an acidic, protein-based conditioner to the hair and leave on for 3 to 5 minutes. Rinse in cool water, and proceed to the neutralizing shampoo.

Frizzy Hair

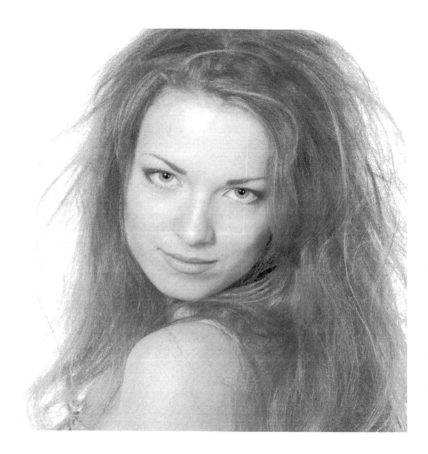

Frizz. The immortal enemy of wanna-be straight- haired chicks as well as those with naturally curly tresses who crave well-defined, popping curls and coils. But—naturally straight-haired folks aren't entirely immune to frizz either. For some, frizz is a natural hair characteristic that plays up considerably when the weather turns for the worse or when hair is exposed to the right amount of shower-time humidity. For others it's a sign of serious damage likely brought about by chemicals and overstyling. While eliminating every single area of frizz is next to impossible, the tips in this section may help you control your frizz a little better.

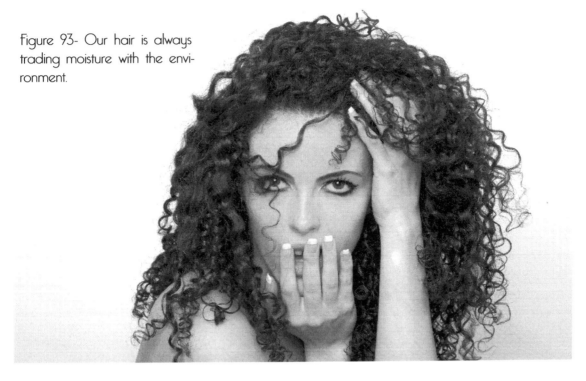

Figure 93- Our hair is always trading moisture with the environment.

Signs & Symptoms

You hear it all the time: Our hair is like a sponge. It is always looking for moisture in the environment to absorb, and when your hair's cuticle is slightly ruffled, either naturally or from damage, the floodgates are open! Moisture easily gets into the hair and causes it to expand, leading to the signs and symptoms below:

• Frizzy, swollen, puffy hair.
• Excessive hair dryness.
• Dull, lackluster hair.

Causes & Triggers

The leading cause of frizz is our hair's 24/7 moisture exchange with the outside environment! The drier or more damaged our hair is, the more frizz it will have. When our hair is porous and dry, it tries to find moisture wherever it can. Most of the time, this moisture is pulled from the air around us—especially when the air is humid.

Products that contain humectants can also affect the way moisture interacts with our hair in different types of weather. For example, when the dew point is fairly high (+60°F range), humectants such as glycerin pull moisture from the air to your hair. When our hair takes in moisture from the air, the hair shaft expands, and hydrogen bonds reform, flattening (or expanding) any style we may have had.

Because naturally wavy and curly hair's cuticle layer has regular areas of lifting, even in the healthiest of heads, some level of frizz is to be expected with this hair type.

The major causes of frizzy hair are:

• Natural shape of the hair fiber (some hair is just naturally frizzy!).
• Heat abuse from hot styling tools including flatirons, curling irons, heated rollers, and blow dryers.

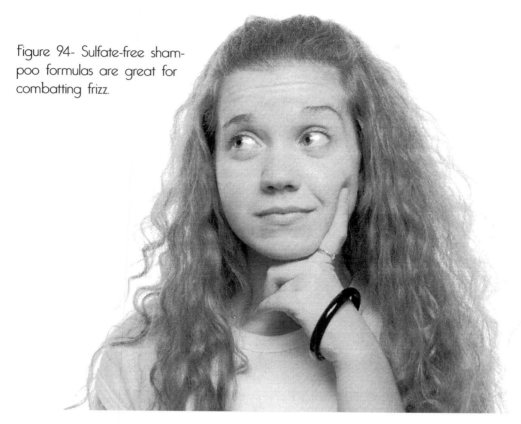

figure 94- Sulfate-free shampoo formulas are great for combatting frizz.

- Increased hair porosity from natural wear to the hair fiber.
- Overprocessing from chemical relaxers, straighteners, and/or permanent colors (i.e., bleaching, highlighting, and lowlighting).
- Cleansing hair in hot water and/or with harsh shampoos.
- Cleansing hair in hard or chlorinated water.
- Exposure to harsh environmental stressors, mainly the sun and wind.
- Using conditioners that are not formulated for your hair type.
- Improper selection of finishing products.

Intervention & Preventing Relapse
Shampoo & Conditioner Power

A good shampoo sets the tone for your entire hair regimen. Start off with a harsh, stripping shampoo, and you'll no doubt have frizzy locks to show for it. Seek out gentle, sulfate-free shampoo formulas whenever possible to stop frizz before it starts. If your shampoo leaves your hair feeling squeaky clean, it is doing way too much. It is very possible to clean the hair without stripping it bare!

Don't underestimate the power of your conditioner, either. Many times, frizzy hair is simply under-conditioned hair that desperately craves moisture! Conditioners hydrate the hair, and also contain emollients that smooth and leave a breathable film on the hair to help prevent frizz. If your hair is thick or naturally curly, try leaving a little conditioner in your hair after you rinse out your shampoo. Leaving a light-weight moisturizing or instant conditioner in the hair after cleansing will help to define your curls and eliminate major frizz.

Reduce Your Hair's Porosity

Porous hair loves to take in moisture from the surrounding environment. If the hair is already properly conditioned prior to venturing outdoors, your chances of trading moisture with the outside air and creating a frizzy situation decrease. Protein treatments will also help you to regulate your hair's porosity. Try the Protein Smoothie from the Special Hair Conditioning & Restoration Treatments section on page 255 (or the olive oil/egg variation, if you need more concentrated strengthening) to add structure to your hair's cuticle layers. The Bentonite Clay Mask (page 251) is also effective at playing down unwanted frizz. If your hair's porosity is kept in check, the moisture trade is even further reduced. For additional porosity control, try a simple Apple-Cider-Vinegar Rinse after your conditioner (see page 250).

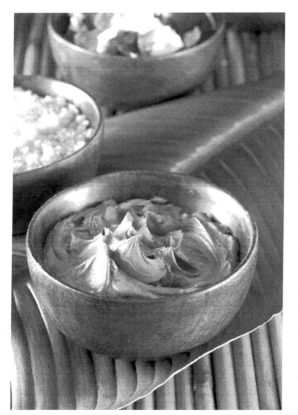

Figure 95- Bentonite clay may help you fight frizz.

Condition the Cuticle with Finishing Products

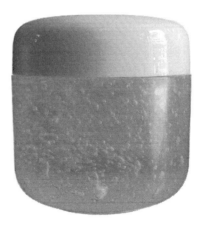

Figure 96- Finishing products may greatly reduce frizz.

Sometimes, you've got to beef up your hair's barriers against the moisture trade. Add a light layer of lubrication to your hair while it is still damp. Serums and light gels are your best frizz-fighting bets. If your hair is fine, lightweight smoothing products in spray, foam, or gel form are better than heavy creams and pomades for combatting frizz without weighing down the hair. Be sure that all products are alcohol-free and are not robbing your hair of moisture.

No other ingredient used in hair care stirs up the masses like silicones. Silicones, such as dimethicone and cyclomethicone, are popular ingredients in conditioners and frizz-busting products because when it comes to blocking moisture entry into the hair from the outside (or preventing heat damage from hot tools)—they are hard to beat. However, for some people, overuse of silicone-based products over time can lead to buildup, hair dryness, and frazzled locks. Some stubborn silicones also require more rigorous shampooing for their removal, which can also lead to drier hair and frizzier end results. Always consider your own hair type and preferences before declaring war against silicones in your hair care. Some people avoid silicones entirely, while others find useful ways to strategically use them in their regimens. There's lots of propaganda out there both for and against them—you'll know where you personally stand after experimenting with your own products.

Frizz-Free Hair Drying

Drying time can make or break your frizz-fighting mission. Carefully blot your hair and avoid rubbing and scrunching a towel through your hair as it dries. A microfiber towel is perfect for frizz-prone wavy, curly and textured hair types and will also protect cuticle orientation

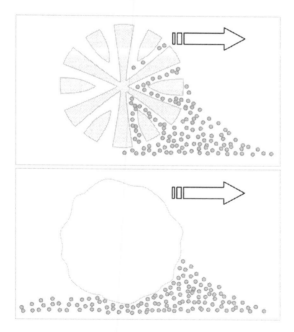

Figure 97- Microfiber towels (top picture) dry the hair quickly by absorbing much more water than conventional towels (bottom picture). Their super-absorbency eliminates the need to ruffle up the hair to dry it.

in straight hair as well. These towels dry hair evenly and quickly without roughing up the hair's cuticles—a process that ultimately leads

to frizz and flyaways. Don't have a microfiber towel on hand? Use a regular T-shirt to absorb excess water from your strands!

Hands Off!

To further reduce frizz in your styling routine, keep your hands out of your hair after you've set it. If you have roller set your hair, ensure that the rollers are pulled taut to avoid puffing and fuzzing of the style, Also, try not to remove rollers before the hair has fully dried. If your hair is being heat straightened, allow the warm hair to cool before combing through it and styling the section. If you are allowing natural curls to set, avoid the temptation to scrunch and touch them. Touching hair during the set will almost always cause more frizz.

Put the Brush Down

Nothing brings on major frizz like a good hair brushing! If your hair is curly or wavy, put the brush down! Brushing curls almost always leads to unwanted frizz and netted, weblike hair. Brushes suitable for detangling (like the Denman) are great, especially for curly girls, but other brushes can increase static and cause your style to assume a mushroom position!

Denman detangling brushes are professional styling brushes that can be purchased in most beauty supply stores or online on Amazon.com for less than ten dollars. These brushes have staggered comblike nylon bristles that are super flexible and easy on the hair. Denman brushes also have removable rows for customized styling. This brush is best used on wet, finger-detangled, wavy or curly hair that is coated with conditioner. When used correctly, it can make detangling a breeze and help define curls and waves. If you find that the brush tangles or breaks your hair, try removing several rows of teeth, or if all else fails, try a shower comb for detangling instead.

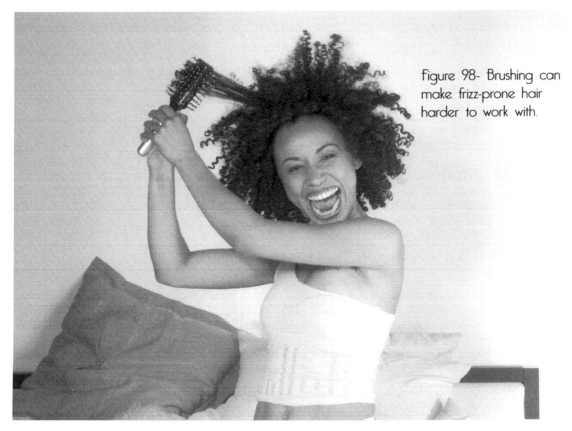

Figure 98- Brushing can make frizz-prone hair harder to work with.

Keep Heat Low

Avoid using heat as much as possible. Heat greatly increases porosity which reduces your hair's ability to keep the right moisture in and the outside humidity out! If using a hair dryer is a must for your hair, use a diffuser or hooded dryer unit to reduce the negative effects of heat.

Trim off the Bad Stuff

If you have frizziness concentrated near the ends of your hair that doesn't improve with cuticle-smoothing treatments, your hair may be due for a maintenance trim. Normal wear and tear can cause split and frayed ends that do not behave well, no matter what products are applied to the hair. Trimming your hair will set the record straight again.

Figure 99- A Denman brush is a great detangler for frizz-prone hair. Denman also makes paddle brushes and other types of brushes for your hair's detangling needs.

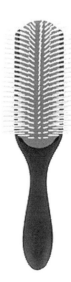

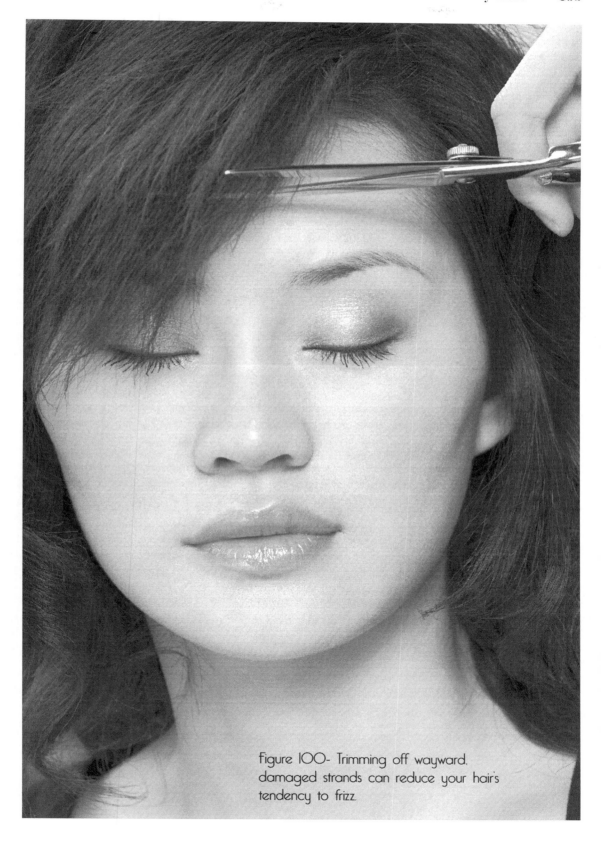

Figure 100- Trimming off wayward, damaged strands can reduce your hair's tendency to frizz.

Graying Hair

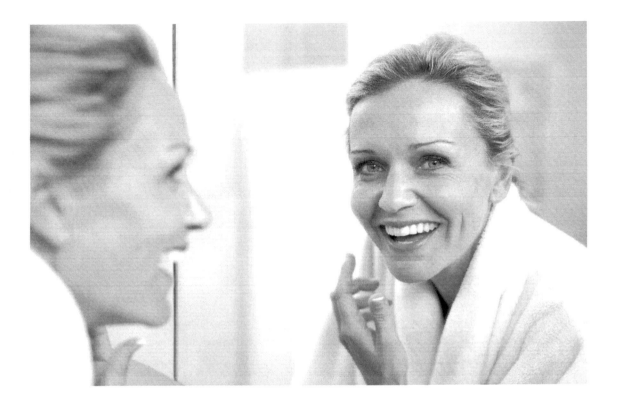

Everyone remembers their "firsts"—the first kiss, the first "real" job, the *first gray hair*. And usually—after the unlucky strand has been plucked out a time or two, and your hair's natural part has been cleverly shifted to disguise the rogue hair—you finally give in and go with the middle-aged flow. Gray hair can either be a blessing or a curse—a sign of wisdom to come or a painful reminder that we're simply getting . . . well, *older*. In the world of gray, maintenance options are often pretty black and white— Camouflage or let the gray come in. Whether you have finally decided to embrace your silver, pearl, or snowy tresses or are trying to survive a few more years without a single silver strand, the tips in this section will help you make peace with your aging hair.

Signs & Symptoms
Although grays can come in at any age (even as early as the teen years), middle age is when silvery shades reign supreme. Signs of gray include the appearance of:

- Gray, wiry strands.
- Hair texture changes, usually from fine or medium to coarse.

Causes & Triggers
First, let's begin with a pretty important fact: There is no such thing as a gray hair! As we get older, the color pigment cells in our hair follicles stop producing color—period. When this happens, the hair shaft begins to grow in clear or white. Contrasted against other hairs on the head (which have not gone completely clear), our eyes perceive the color gray. That's right: Gray is not an actual hair color!

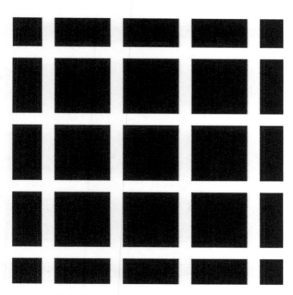

Figure 101- This Hermann Grid demonstrates how we "see" gray hair.

Look at the image in Figure 101. This well-known color illusion is known as the Hermann Grid. No gray was used to create this black and white image, but if you glance at the image, you will see the color gray begin to fill in the little intersections between the large black squares. If you just stare at one intersection at a time, the gray color will disappear and seem to become white. Try it! The same thing happens with your hair. If you focus on one particular hair, you will notice that it is not gray at all! It is indeed clear or white. This is the exact same optical trick our eyes play on us every single time we see a gray-haired person!

So, what ultimately determines when we finally go gray? Genes. You'll likely start graying around the same time as your parents or grandparents. Some studies have shown that race/ethnic background also plays a role in the graying process; those of Caucasian and Asian descent often begin graying in their mid- to late thirties, while those of African descent often begin sometime in the mid-forties. You are considered prematurely gray if more than 50 percent of your hair is gray before age forty.

Besides genes and natural aging, other health-related factors can bring on grays prematurely including vitamin B12 deficiency, thyroid disorders, and even smoking.

Intervention & Preventing Relapse
Beef up on Vitamin B12
The B vitamins, particularly vitamin B12, are especially critical to healthy hair pigmentation and growth. Slack on the B vitamins, and you may start to see silvery strands crop up sooner than you'd planned. Vitamin-B deficiency is rare, but it can affect vegetarians, the elderly, and those with intestinal or liver issues. B vitamins are naturally found in meats and dairy products, so a diet rich in these foods will ensure that you receive the necessary amounts of B vitamins. (Of course, always check with your doctor before starting any diet or vitamin regimen.)

Check Your Thyroid

Our thyroid plays a major role in the health and appearance of our hair. An over- or underactive thyroid can produce grays in addition to altering the hair's overall strength and feel. The thyroid is so powerful that trouble with this gland can even lead to the loss of hair in the outer third of your eyebrow's arch!

Silver Acceptance

Aside from ensuring that your diet is balanced and there are no outstanding health issues, the general consensus is that once the grays come in, they are here to stay. Every decade beyond the age of thirty adds a 10 to 20 percent increased chance of graying, and it can take ten years or more from the first appearance of gray until the entire head is fully gray. There are still no scientifically proven treatments, herbs, supplements, or products that are able to stop the natural graying process, despite the feverish pace at which cosmetic companies are researching these desired "breakthroughs in a bottle." This leaves us with two basic

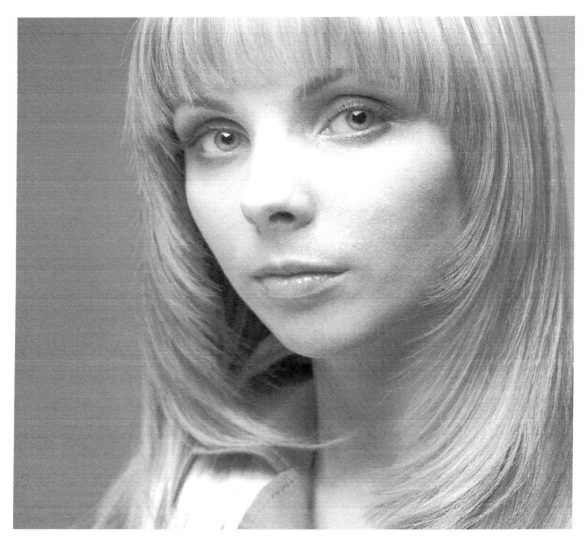

Figure 102- If you are trying to achieve a more youthful look with your graying hair, try bangs. Bangs tend to mask forehead wrinkles and draw attention to the eyes.

interventions for gray hair: Either accept, or camouflage!

If done well, gray (like any other hair color) can be chic, modern, classy, and even sexy! The key to perfectly carrying silver strands is simply ensuring that the hair is well hydrated, conditioned, and cut in a modern style. Mind you, *cut in a modern style* does not necessarily mean "short." Most women go super short on advice that long hair "ages" women after a certain point in time. This one-size-fits-all mentality about hair length and age shouldn't be the final say for you. Long or short, do what makes you feel best! Vibrant, healthy gray strands show that you are confident and in control of your personal style—but dry, ratty, stringy, or frizzy gray hair (or any color for that matter!) looks dated and is a sure way to have concerned friends and family members silently thinking, *Wow, she's really let herself go.* . . . Finally, thinking of gray hair as a bona fide color choice—rather than as a death sentence!—can greatly improve your experience with the process.

Now, if silver acceptance and going gray gracefully are not your cup of tea, here are a few things you can do while you wait for science to come up with the next gray-hair reversal revolution.

Camouflage It!
One thing you should know about grays is that they are super color resistant! Whether you are lightening or darkening your hair, working with grays can be a bit of a challenge—not to mention expensive over time—since any coloring done will need to be touched up regularly.

Newly Graying
If you are new to coloring or not yet completely gray (less than 50 percent), start with a nice semipermanent or deposit-only shade that either matches or is two to three shades lighter than your natural shade. Because they don't contain the chemicals needed to lift color, these colors can't change or brighten your natural hair color, but they will help blend and highlight your lighter, gray strands.

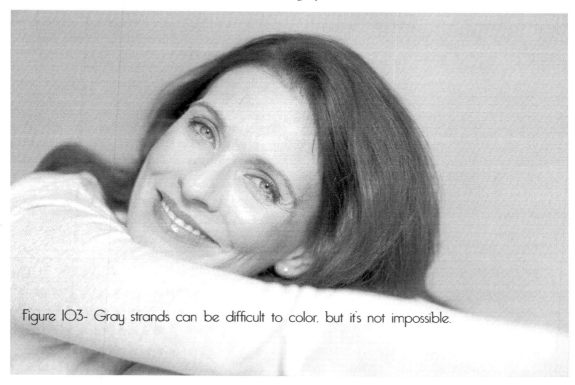

Figure 103- Gray strands can be difficult to color. but it's not impossible.

Steer clear of alcohol- or peroxide-based colors because they will sap moisture from already dry-feeling gray strands. It's also important that you avoid the temptation to rinse out the color prematurely! Leaving the color product on the hair for the full processing time will ensure that the color takes and your gray is covered sufficiently.

To keep your color coverage looking great, use a hair color wand in your natural color to paint and blend incoming new growth. These handy sticks of touch-up color are almost indistinguishable from regular eye mascara wands and work great if you have minimal gray. (In fact, if you are really on a tight budget, use a mascara wand to paint your grays!) Remember to always use color-safe shampoos and conditioners to gently cleanse and condition the hair.

Advanced Graying

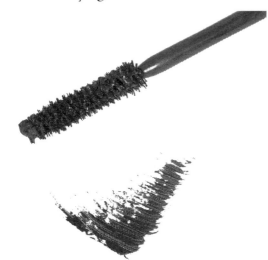

Figure 104- Color wands are perfect for touch-up color applications.

If your hair is more than 50 percent gray, permanent coloring is the best way to go. While many of us can get away with coloring at home in the bathroom with few issues, covering an entire head of gray hair with color is best left to the professionals. Because gray hair tends to be wirier than the naturally colored hair, presoftening the gray prior to coloring may help it accept the color better. Peroxide is a common presoftening agent. You should see a salon for presoftening services if you are inexperienced; again, this is best for those with considerable graying.

Gray hair is often unpredictable and getting natural, even color coverage can be difficult when color-treating. If you are intent on bleaching your graying hair to achieve super-bright, golden shades, you'll definitely want a stylist on hand. Your stylist will ensure that you avoid that telltale *I-don't-know-what- I'm-doing* yellowy color that is so common for gray.

Henna

The trend today is to avoid chemical exposure at all costs. Unfortunately, many commercial hair-color brands contain chemicals that have been linked to (or at least blamed for) some pretty serious health ailments. For those who prefer coloring the natural way, henna is a great option for coloring grays. Henna, on its own, produces a red-orange hair color on gray strands, so if red-orange strands are appealing to you, then go for it! Other plant powders—indigo, for example—can be added to henna to produce deeper, darker hues; but the red tones will always reign supreme once the color begins its natural fadeout. The downside to henna is that achieving a consistent color can be a challenge and an art! The color may be unpredictable from application to application and may vary depending upon the quality of your henna powder. The process is also time-consuming, and if you aren't careful, it can also be rather messy!

NOTE: Always work with body-art quality (BAQ) henna. This is pure henna, free of harmful metallic dyes and additives. If you decide to try henna, only purchase it from reputable

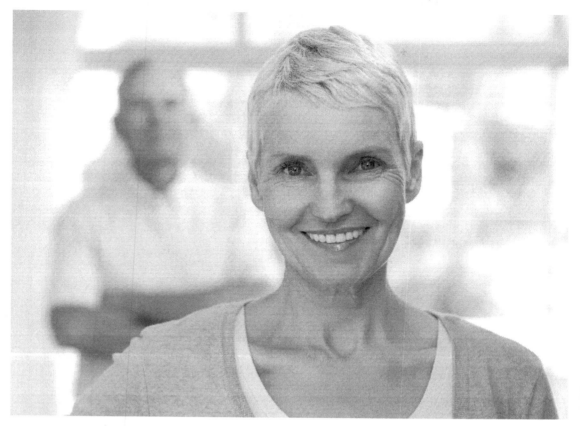

Figure 105- Growing gray can be an interesting challenge.

dealers such as mehandi.com or a trusted local dealer.

Graying Gracefully

While a vast majority of thirty-, forty-, and fifty-somethings choose to color their hair at least initially, there are some who simply have chosen not to fight Mother Nature. Depending on how you are graying, the graying process can be pretty easy or a monumental challenge. Usually, both a mental and physical hair transition will be involved. The more contrast there is between your natural hair color and the gray—or the more concentrated your gray hairs are in a particular region of the scalp—the more challenging it can be to maintain a natural look. There is also an element of time that must be factored into the equation, so be prepared for a bit of a journey as the process toward a "natural look" can take some time to complete.

If you aren't ready to stop coloring your grays cold turkey, a bit of camouflage can also help the graceful graying process. One way to gray gracefully is to simply blend the new growth with a semipermanent color while progressively trimming the ends of the hair to remove the old, fully pigmented hair. Another way to go gray is to simply go for the gusto, and cut the hair into a short style that fully removes the colored hair. This no-fuss method is best for those who don't mind taking drastic measures and for those who are almost completely gray.

Green Hair

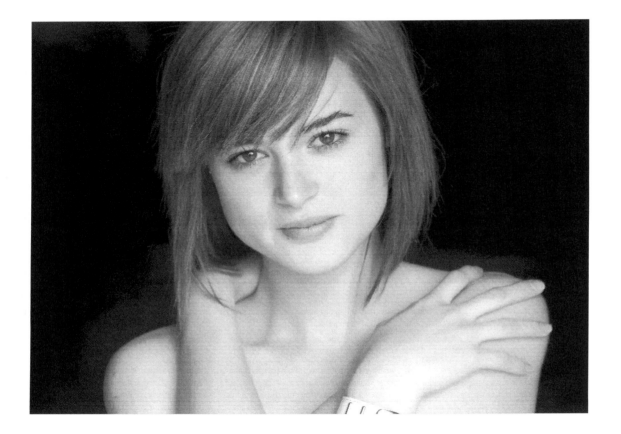

Green hair? While it's rarely a desirable color choice, if your hair is gray, blonde, bleached, or light-colored, you've probably had an experience or two with green- or aquamarine-tinted hair. Green hair can happen to those of us with dark-colored tresses too. If you've ever tried to backtrack and cover a botched, do-it-yourself hair lightening job with a blue-black color rinse, for example, the green may show in certain lighting. But greenish-tinged hair really stands out for those with the lightest natural hair colors. The tips in this section will help you fix your green hair!

Signs & Symptoms

- Greenish tint to light-colored hair strands.
- Excessive hair dryness.
- Dull, lackluster hair.

Causes & Triggers

The most common and perhaps most well-known cause of green highlights is swimming-pool water, but there are several situations that can lead to green hair:

- Swimming-pool water.
- Hard water.
- Botched hair coloring.

Water Woes

Now, most of us associate weird green hair with the chlorine in pool water—but chlorine is actually innocent here. Instead, we should all direct our angst at copper. Yes, copper! While chlorine does have a bleaching effect on the hair, copper is the true cause of green hair that comes from pool water or any other water. Remember those really old copper pennies with the blue-green crust on them? It is the same principle. The copper metal ions bond to your hair's proteins and give off their natural blue-green hue!

But how do we come in contact with copper? Interestingly, copper lurks in some pretty common places. Copper often enters pools and showers when it leaches from copper-piping or is introduced into the water in the form of algae-fighting chemicals that are used to keep the water fresh and clear. Copper can stick to hair, fingernails, skin, and even light-colored bathing suits! Some hair-coloring chemicals can also interact with copper to leave green tints on the hair.

Do-It-Yourself Coloring Mishaps

Hair coloring seems simple enough—choose a shade that you like, pick up a box kit, and go! But if you're blonde, the coloring process may be just a bit trickier. If you aren't familiar with the color rules used in hair care, you can set yourself up for some unintentional green highlights! When happy do-it-yourselfers with blonde or light-colored tresses apply ash or cool base colors to their hair to make it brunette, greenish undertones are often the result.

Intervention & Preventing Relapse

Luckily, preventing and treating green hair is pretty simple.

Chelate Like Nobody's Business!

If you've already fallen victim to copper-induced green hair, never fear! Restoring the hair's normal color is as simple as reaching for shampoo. In order to restore hair to its original color, a chelating shampoo (also called swimmer's shampoo) must be used. (See page 75 for more information on chelating shampoos.) You'll need to thoroughly deep condition your hair following the chelating shampoo, since these shampoos can be really hard on your hair, especially with extended use.

Try an Aspirin Wash

If you do not have a chelating shampoo on hand, try an aspirin wash to counteract the copper. Simply crush and grind up a few aspirin tablets, and add them to your normal shampoo. The

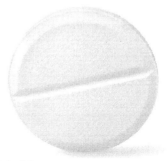

Figure 106- "Aspirin rinsing" can help return hair to its natural shade.

aspirin contain salicylic acid, which helps to neutralize the green-blue copper.

Vinegar Rinsing

We know that vinegar is an excellent stain remover for clothes, hands, and just about anything else—and hair is no exception. Combine ¼ cup of apple cider vinegar (or plain vinegar) with 1 to 1 ½ cups pure water. Pour this mixture over the hair as a final hair rinse after conditioning to restore the hair's natural color and improve hair shine and manageability.

Pre-shampoo the Tomato Way

Not just for removing stubborn skunk odors anymore, tomato juice used as a pre-shampoo treatment may also help to remove the greenish tint from your hair because it acts as a red-based toner. Simply apply tomato juice (or a can of V8 juice) to your hair, massage in, and cover with a plastic shower cap for 15 minutes. Rinse well, and shampoo and condition as normal. If you'd prefer to skip the tomato juice, just pick up a red-based toner product from your local beauty supply store to neutralize the green tones.

Fill It Up!

The best way to combat green hair is to stop it before it ever begins. If swimming caps are not your cup of tea, use the power of water to protect your hair from color-changing madness! Before jumping into the pool, saturate your hair first with pure water. Hair can only absorb so much water, so if it is "full" before you hop into the pool, then the pool water won't be able to affect it as much. As an additional layer of protection,

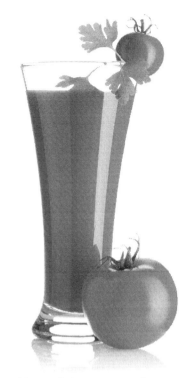

Figure 107- Channel the power of tomato to fix green tresses.

run some conditioner through your hair before getting in the water. When your swim time is up, immediately rinse your hair with pure water.

Talk to Your Stylist

It's great to be adventurous, but some things are best left to the professionals. If you are still determined to color your hair on your own—get a second opinion from your hair stylist before settling on a shade. This may save you from having to return to his or her chair later with algae-colored hair and an even higher corrective hair-coloring service fee!

Hair Loss & Thinning

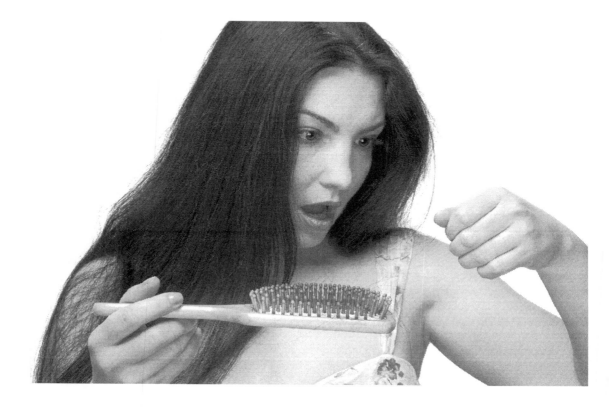

When you look in the mirror, do you see scalp staring back at you? Is your ponytail looking whisper thin? Hair thinning can be a traumatic event for anyone. Hair that was once lush and vibrant may slowly become lank and thin over time. Once a problem associated with men, women too often deal with thinning hair. Problems can start as early as the teen years for some individuals; however, for most people, hair thinning becomes most pronounced in the thirties and forties. By age forty, nearly half of adults will have experienced some thinning. In the United States alone, roughly 30 million women suffer from some form of hair loss or hair thinning. The tips in this section, with your doctor's approval, will help you understand and fight hair thinning and loss.

Signs & Symptoms

On a healthy scalp, our hairs shed day in and day out, but these shed hairs are normally replaced by newly emerging hairs within a few weeks. Most people normally shed fifty to one hundred hairs a day. This delicate process typically affects less than 10 percent of the hairs on a head at one time, so the effects of this shedding remain unseen in the midst of the other actively growing hairs. Hair thinning typically occurs before total hair loss. Common signs and symptoms of hair loss and thinning include:

- Increasingly finer hair strands over time.
- Increasing areas of scalp exposure.

Causes & Triggers

As we get older, there are some pretty interesting changes that occur in our hair follicles' growing phases. The length of time our hair actually spends growing gets shorter and shorter—and over time, the percentage of hairs that are actively growing begins to decrease. With more hairs in the resting phase, the number of hairs that shed slowly begins to increase over time. The new hairs that grow in their place become noticeably thinner as the follicle also starts to shrink in size. Eventually the follicle gets so small that it can no longer produce hair.

Hair Loss

| Normal hair follicle | Follicle shrinking causing hair thinning | Small follicle unable to grow new hair |

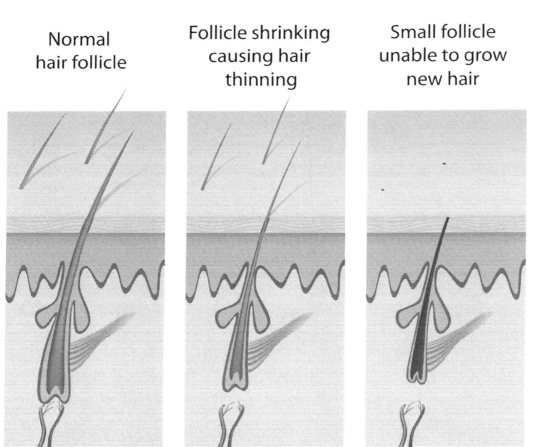

Figure 108- To understand hair loss, notice how follicle size diminishes over time.

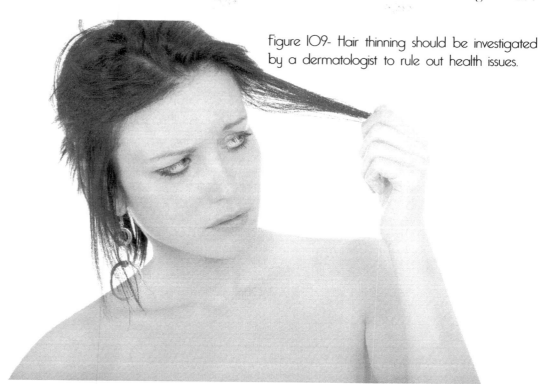

Figure 109- Hair thinning should be investigated by a dermatologist to rule out health issues.

Unfortunately, despite advances in our understanding of hair loss and hair thinning, these processes are still largely misunderstood—although many positive theories have been touted over the years. The top hair loss culprits, as currently understood, are

- Hormonal changes (puberty, pregnancy, menopause).
- Genetics.
- Severe illness or hair/scalp trauma.
- Low-iron diet.
- Thyroid issues and thyroid medications.
- High stress.
- Nutritional problems/fad dieting.
- Medications/surgeries.
- Overworking/overstyling the hair.

Hormones

If you are experiencing abnormal hair loss that isn't letting up, have your hormone levels checked. Hormones control a great deal of what a hair follicle can and cannot do. Certain hormones—typically the male hormones (androgens)—reduce the hair-growing power of the follicles on the scalp. This is why men tend to bald younger, faster, and more substantially than women of a similar age. The estrogens, or female hormones, tend to promote hair growth and protect the hair follicles against the effects of androgens. We can easily see the power of estrogen at work during pregnancy and menopause. In pregnancy, when estrogen levels are at their peak, the hair flourishes and rarely sheds. In menopause, however, when estrogen levels naturally taper off, thinning or balding of the hair is common.

Genetics

About 95 percent of men and 70 percent of women will have thinning as a result of androgenic alopecia, an inherited form of hair loss. This form of hair loss can be inherited from either the mother's or the father's side of the family and may also be related to a sensitivity to certain hormones in the body. It's not uncommon for this form of thinning to skip generations.

Stress & Illness

In addition to estrogen, women also have low amounts of "male hormones" (testosterone), which can increase under periods of high stress. This increase in male hormones can negatively affect hair growth and lead to hair loss.

Health issues such as PCOS (polycystic ovarian syndrome) and thyroid disorders (especially overactive thyroid) can also affect hormone levels in the body, which may lead to hair loss.

High fever and infection can also lead to hair loss a few weeks or months out from the actual illness.

Nutritional Problems

Nutritional deficiencies and eating disorders such as anorexia, bulimia, and fad dieting may also cause temporary hair loss and profuse thinning.

Medications/Surgeries

Hair loss can also be a side effect of some medications that are used to treat other health

When It's Time to See Your Doctor

The cause of your hair loss and/or thinning should be thoroughly investigated by a licensed dermatologist for an official diagnosis before you seek treatment. Although some scientifically proven treatments for hair loss and hair thinning are available over the counter without a prescription, a proper diagnosis should always be sought from an experienced practitioner before embarking on any treatment regimen. Your dermatologist will be able to suggest treatments for hair loss and thinning that are suitable for your situation.

conditions. Some thyroid medications and even oral contraceptives (birth control pills) can trigger hair loss in some people.

Overworking/Overstyling the Hair

High-stress and high-tension styling of the hair can lead to traction alopecia, another medical form of hair loss. Traction alopecia is reversible in its early stages, but if the damaging styling practices are not stopped, hair loss eventually becomes permanent. (See Alopecia, page 104.)

Improper use of chemical treatments such as relaxers, straighteners, perms, and bleaches can also cause direct hair loss.

Intervention & Preventing Relapse

Remember that thinning and balding after the age of forty or fifty is a normal part of the aging process—and this process actually starts over a period of many years before it ever becomes noticeable. Fortunately, advances in scientific research have provided us with several scientifically proven treatments for hair loss and hair thinning. Product manufacturers have also formulated a wide variety of treatments (some great, some not so great) for treating the condition.

Cosmetic Treatments for Hair Thinning

If you are in the early stages of thinning or simply want to avoid medications and treatments, the following cosmetic fixes can work for your thinning hair. Unlike medical treatments, which must work at the follicle level, these methods work at the shaft level by temporarily plumping up individual strands. Except for hair coloring, results will only last from one wash to the next in most cases.

Color It!

Not only does coloring thinning hair add dimension to your tresses, but hair color treatments can also temporarily thicken or plump up your individual hair strands, giving the illusion of fuller hair. While bleaching can also improve the thickness of your hair, it will also inflict considerable damage in the process. Stick with semipermanent and other temporary types of color.

Volumize It!

Store shelves are full of products that promise to volumize and add body to thinning or very fine hair. These products are formulated with light proteins to plump up the hair, and light conditioning agents to add smoothness to the fiber. After-conditioner mousses and foams can be applied to the root area for lift and additional volume.

Keratin Fiber Treatments?

A recent innovation to help counter hair loss involves the use of "keratin fibers" to disguise hair thinning problems. Popular keratin-fiber brands include products such as *Toppik*, *Xfusion*, and *Nanogen*—which essentially resemble dust in a shaker. These treatments come in a variety of colors and thicknesses and are durable enough to stand up to sweat, wind, and even light rain. Microscopic keratin hair fibers are sprinkled onto thinning areas and bind (using static electricity) to the existing hair, giving it a naturally fuller appearance. Some keratin-fiber treatments can even bind to the faint, colorless hairs that may still be present on scalps that otherwise appear to be bald.

The cons? Treatments generally last for only one shampoo, and some users complain that the fibers, while mostly invisible indoors, are easily detectable in sunlight. For those with more complete hair loss, the fibers may simply coat the scalp rather than accentuate remaining hairs. There are also claims that some of the products are not as waterproof as their manufacturers suggest along with horror stories about the products washing out and running down users' faces in the rain.

Check with your dermatologist for more information on these products, and to see if they are right for you.

Medical Treatments for Hair Thinning & Loss

If cosmetic, body-building tricks do not work well for you, your doctor may be able to prescribe medications to work on your hair from below the scalp at the follicle level. Each hair-loss treatment must be used diligently over the prescribed period of time before initial growth results materialize. Once regrowth has occurred, each hair loss and hair thinning treatment must be continued *indefinitely* in order to maintain results. As of this writing, science has simply not provided us with a viable permanent solution or treatment for hair loss problems.

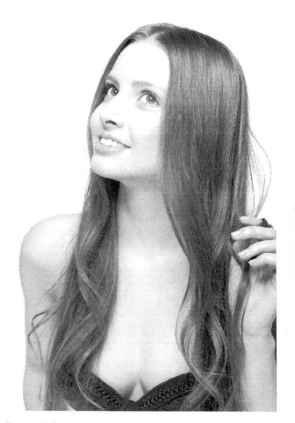

Figure 110- Don't underestimate the power of volumizing shampoo to thicken up the hair.

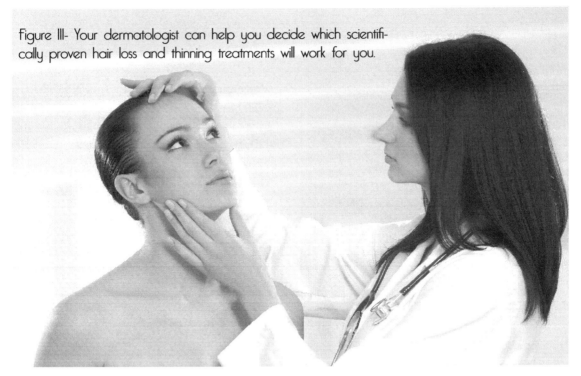

Figure III- Your dermatologist can help you decide which scientifically proven hair loss and thinning treatments will work for you.

Hormone Replacement Therapy

Hormone replacement therapy (HRT) is a common treatment for women with hair loss. HRT helps to replenish hormone levels, particularly estrogens, to levels that were common before menopause. Hormone replacement should be discussed thoroughly with your primary-care physician as it is not without its side effects and risks. Some treatment plans are more hair friendly than others, and your doctor can help you sort through your options.

Minoxidil

Minoxidil is perhaps the most well-known, scientifically proven treatment for hair loss and hair thinning. It has even been shown to grow hair in the ears and in other unintended places! It is the active ingredient in *Rogaine (Regaine, outside the U.S.)*, a popular shampoo for hair loss.

Hair loss and hair thinning treatments containing minoxidil take three to four months of regular use before any hair regrowth results show.

Unfortunately, like most other scientifically proven treatments for hair loss, all newly regrown hair falls out once the medication is stopped. Finally, hair loss treatments containing minoxidil have been shown to actually cause hair loss in some individuals. It is not guaranteed that this hair loss will be compensated for by new hair while continuing to use minoxidil. Do proceed with caution.

Finasteride

Finasteride, the active ingredient in *Propecia* (a popular hair loss prescription medication), is a scientifically proven treatment for hair loss and thinning. Finasteride is very similar to minoxidil and is used to treat male pattern hair loss. Hair loss and hair thinning generally return six to twelve months after discontinuing finasteride.

Finasteride works best on forms of hair loss and thinning that occur in the crown and frontal hairline regions of the scalp. While the treatment is rather effective in men, to date, finasteride has not been proven to be as effective in women—although it is still prescribed for women in some cases. Hair loss and hair thinning treatments containing this ingredient are best for women who are beyond childbearing age. Products containing finasteride should never be used or handled by pregnant women or those who are planning to become pregnant, as it has been known to cause birth defects in developing male fetuses.

Cortisone Injections

Cortisone injections are scientifically proven hair loss treatments that are injected directly into the scalp tissue at the problem site. These scalp injections are especially recommended for hair loss and thinning caused by autoimmune diseases such as lupus or alopecia areata. Unfortunately, any new hair grown through the scalp injection treatment is lost once treatment ends. Cortisone treatments can be administered in pill or topical ointment forms, but the best results typically come from injection treatments.

Essential Oils

Although essential oils are not officially considered scientific treatments for hair loss and thinning, promising studies have been conducted on their validity as effective treatments for these conditions. Many essential oils have stimulating effects on the hair follicles and skin. When massaged into the scalp, oils such as peppermint, rosemary, and thyme work wonderfully as therapies to stimulate and encourage healthy blood flow to the hair follicles in the region. Whether this stimulation *truly* encourages hair growth, however, remains to be seen.

Try massaging your scalp several times per week with a mixture of 3 drops of peppermint oil mixed with 3 to 4 tablespoons of olive or jojoba oil. Allow the mixture to absorb into the scalp for 10 to 15 minutes, and then shampoo the treatment out. You might also try adding just 3 to 5 drops of peppermint oil or rosemary oil to your shampoo for additional scalp invigoration. If the hair follicles have not started to shrink and are still capable of producing hair, this flow of nutrients may help to trigger hair regrowth in some cases.

Head Lice

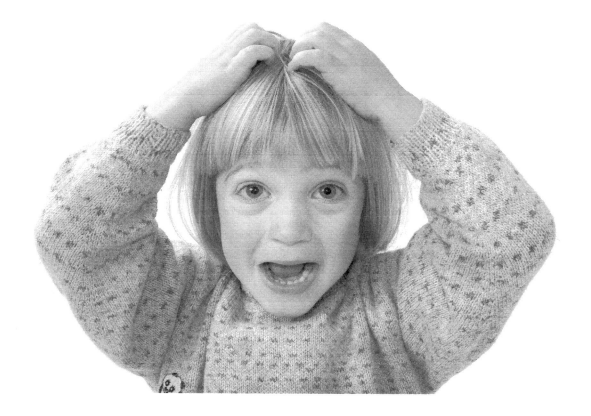

No one invites these six-legged critters to summer camps, sleepovers, and other major childhood get-togethers—but each year, millions of children under the age of twelve are infested with lice. Lice are tiny, wingless insects that live on the hair and scalp. These insects prefer the warmth of the scalp to other parts of the body, and frequently choose the nape area as a favorite nesting spot! Although nearly anyone who comes in contact with lice can be infested, lice are more common in small children than in adults and in girls more than in boys. They aren't dangerous, but they are extremely contagious. One infested child can quickly spread the condition through a classroom. The tips in this section will help you get this six-legged problem under control and avoid becoming a victim yourself!

Signs & Symptoms

Head lice are very small and can be hard to see with the naked eye. To check for lice: Put on a pair of protective gloves and carefully part the hair in small sections under bright lighting. The top of the child's neck and ears are the most common places for nits, or louse eggs, to appear. Signs and symptoms of infestation include:

- Intense scratching.
- Small, red bumps or bites especially on the ears and nape.
- Tiny yellow, tan, or brown specks near the scalp area. These are louse eggs, and they can often look like extremely stubborn dandruff. The eggs are nearly impossible to scratch or brush out and this is what often quickly distinguishes them from regular dandruff. It's more common to see these eggs than live lice crawling around.
- Adult lice and nymphs (developing lice). Gray/tan insects, roughly the size of a sesame seed.

Adult lice live for about a month and lay seven to ten eggs each day. These eggs hatch about one to two weeks after they're laid. The earlier the infestation is caught, the easier it is to clear up.

Causes & Triggers

Lice are spread by contact with an affected person, and they are rarely a sign of poor hygiene. In fact, lice prefer clean hair because it's easier to cling to! Anyone can get them. You can get head lice if you:

- Share hats, clothing, towels, brushes, combs, or other personal items belonging to someone who has had lice.

Intervention & Preventing Relapse

If you or your child is diagnosed with head lice, don't panic. Treating an outbreak is pretty

When It's Time to See Your Doctor

If your child is scratching his/her head constantly and complaining of an intense scalp itch that won't go away, the problem may be lice. In most cases, this is not a serious medical issue and can be treated with over-the-counter medication. If over-the-counter treatments for lice do not work, the condition may require treatment by a physician. Intense scratching can lead to a bacterial infection if not treated. Because lice are so easily spread from person to person, always notify your child's school officials immediately if your child has been diagnosed with head lice.

straightforward these days. The sooner the lice are detected and treated, the better.

Shampoo Regimen

Finding safe, natural remedies for lice is pretty important since children tend to use these products more than anyone else. There are several over-the-counter lotions, rinses, and shampoos that can combat louse infestation.

Neem oil-based shampoos have been shown to be effective against lice in some sufferers. They help to prevent head lice from developing properly—

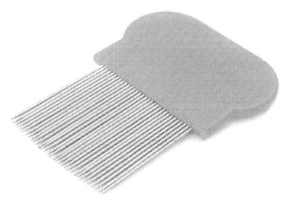

Figure 112- Typical nit comb.

which works especially well against nits and younger lice. While neem-based products do not kill lice right away, they do work over time (one or two days). Tea tree oil-based products, although less effective, are also common treatments for lice. It's not uncommon to find neem and tea tree together in scalp products like these.

Medicated products containing I percent permethrin or 0.5 percent malathion in isopropanol are also common louse-fighting products. Malathion-based products are often used for resistant or hard-to-fight louse infestations. However, since this active ingredient also contains some warnings for use, please seek medical attention before incorporating it into your shampoo regimen.

To combat lice, simply rinse the hair and pat it dry. Apply the shampoo, rinse or lotion and allow it to sit undisturbed on the hair and scalp for ten minutes (or the amount of time specified by the manufacturer). Rinse thoroughly, and proceed with the conditioning phase as necessary.

Since these treatments are not always 100 percent effective and can leave some stray nits, it's always a good idea to follow treatment with a nit comb. Nit combs can be purchased at your local drug store. We will talk about these more, a bit later.

Remove the Nits (Eggs)

If you would rather not use pesticides or special products to treat lice, then a regular cleansing with your favorite shampoo followed by conditioner is an effective, pesticide-free way to get the job done— if used along with a nit comb. If you've ever tried to remove nits from the hair, you know firsthand that it's no easy task! Lice move quickly and use a cement-like glue to ensure that their eggs stay attached firmly to the hair shaft, no matter how active the elementary-school host! Fortunately, nit combs with their

extremely closely-spaced metal teeth are perfect for catching lice and their eggs. To make egg removal a breeze:

1. Oil the hair with olive oil or another oil of your choice and detangle with a large comb.
2. Separate the hair and work it into small sections to prepare for the nit comb.
3. Go through each section with the nit comb until the nits have been completely removed.
4. Remove the hair from the comb and clean it out with a piece of tissue. Discard the tissue by flushing it down the toilet. Clean the nit comb by placing it in a bowl of hot, soapy water before moving on to the next section.
5. Pin your cleared sections out of the way and repeat the combing until the entire head has been combed.
6. Shampoo the hair with a clarifying shampoo and condition the hair as normal.

Comb the hair with the nit comb once or twice per day for three days at a time, or as directed. Alternatively, you may use the nit comb following each regular hair-washing and conditioning session.

Wash Affected Linens & Clothing

Lice are able to live off the scalp for up to two days. To prevent lice from spreading to others, or from re-infesting your child, wash all clothes and bed linens in hot water with detergent. Carpets in affected areas should be vacuumed regularly as well. Nit combs should be placed in hot, soapy water for 10 to 15 minutes or boiled (if they are the sturdier variety).

Implement a No-Sharing Policy

We teach our kids to share their toys and pretty much everything else, but in the case of personal items such as combs, brushes, hats and scarves, we should draw a line. Classrooms can be unavoidably close living quarters during the day, with shared coat and backpack hooks, racks, and cubbies. If lice are a problem in your child's classroom, ask the teacher to space out the children's belongings to prevent cross-infestation.

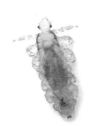
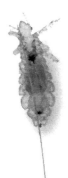
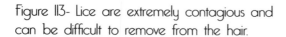

Figure 113- Lice are extremely contagious and can be difficult to remove from the hair.

Heat Damage

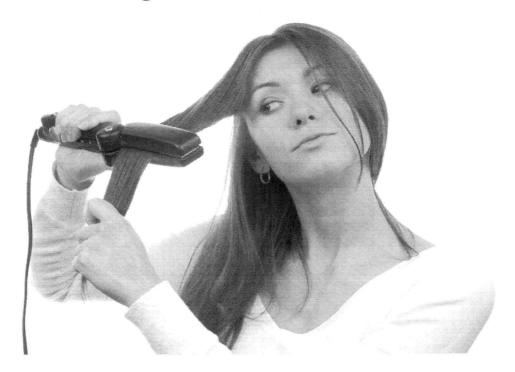

Curly hair that won't revert back to curly, wavy hair that just hangs limp, and straight hair that smells like, well, smoke: These are just some of the hallmarks of heat damage. Thanks to the quick styling highs we get from our blow dryers, curling irons, and straighteners, heat damage is one of the most common causes of hair damage and hair frustration. Some of us can get away with rampant heat use much longer than others, but in the end, excessive heat use always leads to two things: split ends and hair breakage. The tips in this section will help you get your heat-stressed hair under control.

Signs & Symptoms

Did you know that our hair burns at roughly the same temperature as paper (233°C or 451.4°F)? But hair that is already in trouble can burn or scorch at even lower temperatures than this. Common signs and symptoms of heat damage are:

- Excessive hair dryness.
- Thin, splitting ends.
- Increased flyaways.
- Rampant hair breakage.
- Curls that do not return, even after wetting.
- Lightened (reddened) hair color.

The big problem with heat damage is that it is often unnoticeable at first. The first styling session typically is not what does people in. In fact, most of us indulge in heat use for long periods of time (sometimes years) before ever realizing just what it has done to our hair. But the small damaging effects of heat use are cumulative. Heat destroys important structural bonds in the hair fiber, which can permanently straighten wavy and curly hair or severely lengthen out the curl pattern in an unpredictable way. When the hair is rewet (which would normally bring waves and curls back to life), the hair just hangs there, curly in some spots but eerily straight and stringy in others. Heat damage can affect those with straight hair, too. Dryness, splitting, and uneven color from roots to ends are common telltale signs that straight hair has been given more heat than it can handle.

Causes & Triggers

Repeated heat use and straightening disrupts the protein structure of hair and wears away at our hair's protective cuticle layers. Heat also destroys important hydrogen bonds in the hair, which can lead to a loss of curl pattern for those with naturally curly hair and to a loss of moisture for all users, regardless of hair type. The causes of heat damage are pretty straightforward. Your heated appliance (straightener, curling iron, hot rollers, steamer) was simply hotter than your hair could handle— simple as that!

Intervention & Preventing Relapse
Protect before Styling With Heat

Heat protection starts well before your flatiron, hot curler, or blow dryer ever touches your hair. Hair is best protected from heat damage when it has been properly deep conditioned with both moisture and protein-based conditioners just prior to heat use. Poorly moisturized hair heats rapidly and is damaged more easily. A heat-protectant spray, lotion, or serum will also help dissipate the heat through your hair slowly and in an even, controlled manner. Silicone-based products are the ultimate in heat protection—

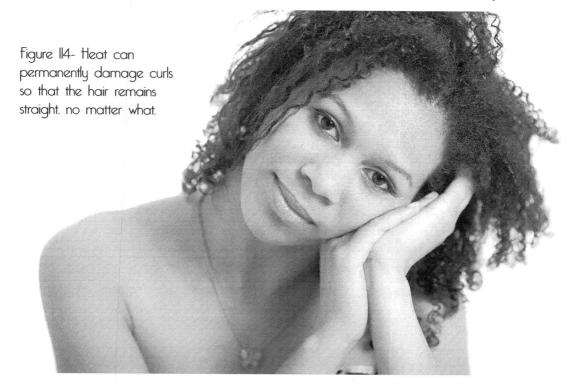

Figure 114- Heat can permanently damage curls so that the hair remains straight. no matter what.

they are a must-have for any serious heat users. While they can't protect you 100 percent from your heat, using heat without them is asking for trouble!

Make Your Appliances Heat Friendly

If you are straightening or hot curling the hair, be sure that your appliance is clear of crusty hair-product residues. The gunk between the plates can harden when dry and scratch and damage your hair. For best results with blow drying, use your dryer's diffuser attachment or a hooded dryer to dry the hair with less damage. Keep all heat appliances moving, and avoid lingering too long on any one section of hair.

To avoid frying your hair, keep your heat appliances dialed down to the lowest heat setting that still allows you to achieve your styling goals. Since heat tolerances vary, know your limits! Work with flatirons and straighteners that have real, dedicated temperature controls that give a specific temperature reading in degrees—not just an on/off, 10-15-20, or high/low switch—so that you can control the heat.

Establish a Heat Schedule that Works for You

Here, you will have to use your best judgment. Some of us have strands of steel that can tolerate regular heat use, while others of us have to use heat sparingly to preserve our tresses. It is not difficult to determine where you fall. If you are intent on using heat more often than several times per week, you will always get the best results if your hair is shoulder length or shorter, medium to coarse textured, naturally straight or wavy, and not chemically treated. Tweaking any of those variables will land you in Hair Care Rehab!

If Your Hair Is Heat Damaged

Here are some tips for working with already damaged hair:

Go on a Heat Hiatus

Carefully unplug and put away your heated styling tools until you have your heat damage under control! Restoring the hair after heat damage can take several weeks of regular and serious conditioning efforts. Eliminate all sources of heat except hooded dryer heat for deep

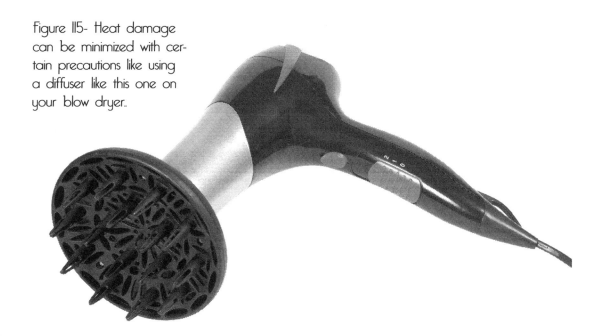

Figure 115- Heat damage can be minimized with certain precautions like using a diffuser like this one on your blow dryer.

conditioning or styling to set the hair on the path to recovery.

Remember, heat-damaged hair will only get worse with additional heat styling. Nothing gets hair back on track like working with your natural hair texture for a change! But if a complete heat hiatus is too difficult for you, simply eliminate heat that you *can* live without in your regimen. For example, air dry your hair in loose braids and touch up with a flatiron— or blow dry with a diffuser, but skip the hot-curling step afterward.

Try a Protein Treatment

Please step away from the appliances and reconstruct your hair with protein! The protein strengthening treatments and products in the Outpatient Therapy section of this book work well for bringing heat-damaged tresses back to life. Keep in mind that if the heat damage is pretty extensive, the hair may not fully recover. Always follow strengthening products with appropriate moisturizing deep conditioners to put elasticity back in the hair.

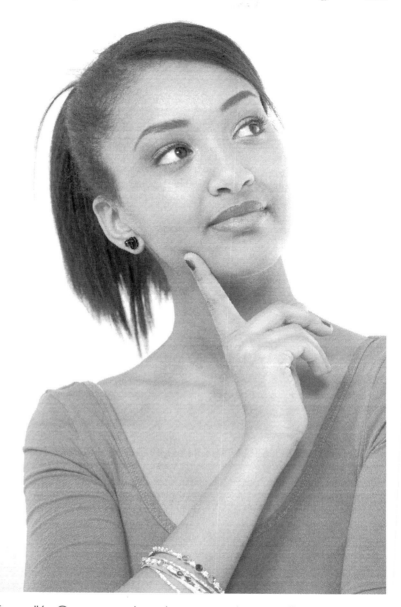

Figure 116- Going on a heat hiatus can dramatically improve the appearance and condition of your hair.

intense, you'll need a more invasive procedure! If your hair still doesn't look better after a few weeks of treatment with moisture and protein, slowly trim out the heat-damaged sections of hair.

Break out the Scissors

While treating the hair with protein usually perks up wayward strands, if the damage is too

Oily Hair

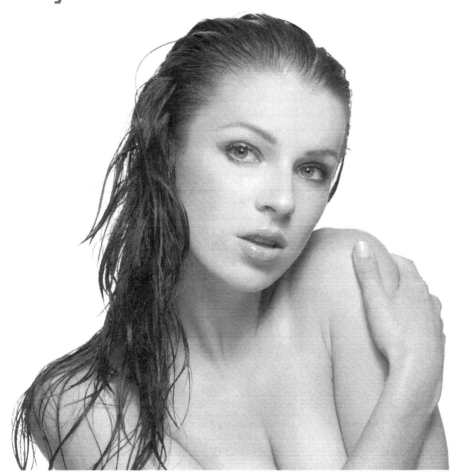

It can be a tough world out there if you have oily hair. Dry, parched hair captivates more hearts, minds, and research dollars in the beauty-product industry than any other hair type. The slew of ultra-rich, super-thick moisturizing products on the market today—*that work so exceptionally well for those with parched tresses*—leaves those will oily hair greasier than ever! Once a problem associated with puberty, many older adults are finding that they are still no match for oil glands that have kicked into high gear! If your hair is short, or naturally straight or wavy—your locks are even more prone to oil slicks! Fortunately, whether you're a teenager or someone who left behind the teen years many moons ago, the tips in this section may help you reach a truce with your oily strands!

Signs & Symptoms

- Oily scalp and hair (or oily scalp with dry ends).
- Limp, lank hair.
- Skin breakouts, especially in places where hair makes contact with the face.

Causes & Triggers

Did you know that every single hair comes with its own set of oil glands? If your hair is oily, you are probably fully aware of each and every one of them! These glands nourish and coat the hair with a protective layer of oil as it grows from the scalp.

But occasionally, the oil-production process goes into overdrive, either naturally or because we're adding more product to our hair than is needed. If your hair is naturally fine, you are more likely to have oily hair. Why? Because you tend to have more hair per square inch of scalp than those with thicker strands—more hair equals more oil glands! Since each hair strand is small, it doesn't take much time to cover them. So—what started out as bouncy, behavin' hair at 8:30 A.M. can quickly disintegrate into flat, greasy hair by 3 P.M.!

The major causes of oily hair are:

- Overactive oil glands (genetic).
- Overuse of products such as oils and serums.
- Using a conditioner product that is too heavy or too rich in oils for your hair type.
- Poor diet, lack of B vitamins.
- Medication.

Intervention & Preventing Relapse
Shampoo Regimen

You probably know better than anyone else that oily hair may need more cleansing than other hair types. A gentle daily rinsing and/

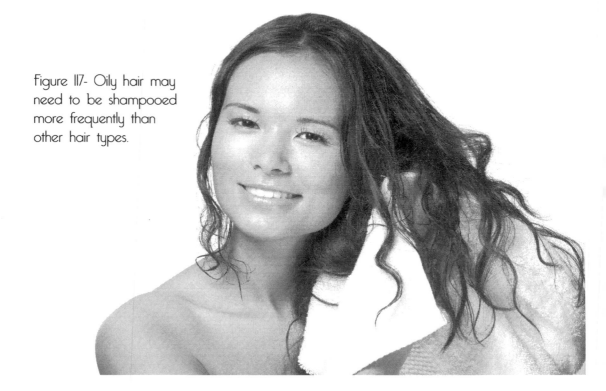

Figure 117- Oily hair may need to be shampooed more frequently than other hair types.

or shampoo will keep excessive natural oils at bay. Look for clear shampoos. These won't contain the extra emollients and oils that will only make your situation worse! Clarifying the hair once a week will also keep the oil under control.

If you have an oily scalp and oily hair near the roots that tends to fall flat as the days wear on, then a dry shampoo may be another alternative for you. These oil-absorbing shampoos freshen up the hair and scalp and help buy you a few more days between regular wet shampooings. Dry shampoos come in powders, sprays, and foams and are applied to the roots and scalp. Today's formulas will lightly clean without overdrying your hair. These shampoos can really come to the rescue in a crunch situation! Try the Dry Cocoa Shampoo recipe (see Special Hair Conditioning & Restoration Treatments, page 252), or for some great commercial dry-shampoo options, see On the Shelf! (page 268).

Conditioner?

If your hair is oily, you may not need a conditioner at every single cleansing. Yes, it might sound odd to those of us who've grown up thinking of shampoo and conditioner as an inseparable duo—but it's all about finding the balance that is right for your hair's unique situation. If your hair detangles easily after you've cleansed it with shampoo, skipping the traditional conditioner step may work for you. If you do use conditioner, simply focus the product along the length and ends of the hair to avoid pesky oil and product buildup near the scalp.

For more information on oily hair issues, check out the section on **Fine, Limp Hair**, page 154.

Psoriasis

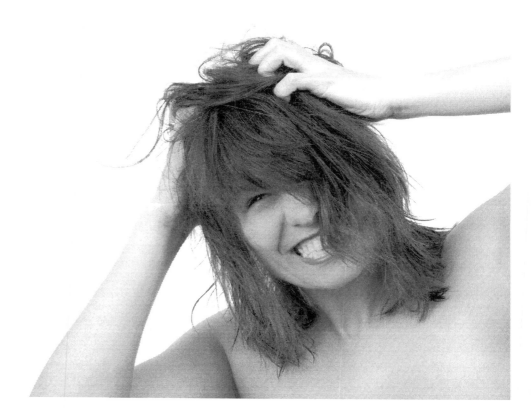

If you think dandruff is bad, try psoriasis on for size! This flaky, itchy scalp condition is simply dandruff gone into overdrive. On a typical scalp, skin cells go through their life cycles and shed in just a month's time. This shedding process happens so smoothly that we rarely notice it. But psoriasis speeds up the process. Psoriasis sufferers have skin cells that grow, mature, and shed five to seven times faster than normal. Because these cells are pumped out so quickly, the body isn't able to remove them fast enough. What do we get? Patches of flaky skin cells that can be layers thick on the scalp. Fortunately, the tips in this section, used with your dermatologist's approval, may help you get your psoriasis under control.

Signs & Symptoms

Psoriasis affects nearly 7 million people in the United States alone. Although the condition can occur just about anywhere on the body, half of all people with psoriasis have it on the scalp. Those between the ages of fifteen and thirty-five are most likely to be affected by this skin condition. Common symptoms include:

- Itchy, large, loose white or silvery flakes on the scalp.
- Bright red patches of dry skin.
- Scaling and crusting made up of hard, super adherent flakes.

Causes & Triggers

So, what causes the skin to produce more and more unneeded skin at such an incredible rate? Unfortunately, scientists have not been able to pinpoint the exact cause of scalp psoriasis. Although the true cause is anyone's guess, here are some commonly cited causes:

- Weak immune system.
- Genetics.
- Stress.
- Poor elimination of body toxins.

Weak Immune System

A weakened immune system is a commonly cited trigger of psoriasis flare-ups. A miscommunication within the body causes the immune system to produce lots of new skin cells when they aren't needed. These cells pile up and create a thick mass many layers thick that can become tender and red. Some researchers propose that psoriasis is triggered when the body's toxins are eliminated through the skin rather than through the liver or kidneys, where they should be.

Genetics

If a family member suffers from psoriasis, you may be at greater risk for the condition. Preliminary research suggests that genetic predisposition plays a role in who gets psoriasis.

Stress & Other Health Conditions

Stress, skin injuries, allergies, alcohol abuse, inadequate sunlight, and some heart medications may also be to blame for psoriasis. Since cases of psoriasis are lower in countries where dietary fat intake is also relatively low, diet is also considered to be an instigator.

When It's Time to See Your Doctor
If you think you may have scalp psoriasis, see a dermatologist for diagnosis. Very often, scalp flaking and scaling conditions mimic one another. Dandruff can look like psoriasis, and seborrheic dermatitis can look like dandruff, for example. Because psoriasis often occurs as a symptom of other health problems, such as diabetes and heart disease, it is important to catch it quickly. If your psoriasis condition worsens, seek medical attention.

What's the Difference between Dandruff & Scalp Psoriasis?

Psoriasis and dandruff both feature flakes and itching, but psoriasis flakes tend to be much larger than standard dandruff flakes. These larger flakes are also less likely to just flake off. Psoriasis also does not limit itself to the scalp area, and often affects other areas of the body.

Intervention & Preventing Relapse
Shampoo Therapy

While there is no real cure for psoriasis, several over-the-counter and prescription options exist for managing the condition. *Nizoral* shampoo, an effective topical treatment against psoriasis, is available in most drug stores without a prescription. Psoriasis, unfortunately, tends to flare up again when shampoo treatment ends.

Skip the Blow Dryer

Blow drying the hair can easily dry out the skin, aggravating flaking. Allow the hair to air dry after cleansing and conditioning when possible.

Make Dietary Changes

Psoriasis is like almost every other skin ailment—it often responds well to changes in our diet. For best results, increase the percentage of raw fruits (excluding citrus fruits such as oranges, grapefruits, lemons, and limes) and vegetables in your diet. Increase your water intake, and pay close attention to your fat intake. Fried, fatty foods and citrus fruits may aggravate psoriasis-prone skin. Increasing fiber in your diet will help ensure that wastes and toxins are properly eliminated from your body.

Sunlight Therapy

Giving your scalp a little sun may provide relief from psoriasis because the sun helps to quickly turn over skin cells before they accumulate in thick patches. Direct sun therapy (or heliotherapy) works best for psoriasis sufferers when it is combined with other treatments, and if it is done several times each day for short exposure times of 5 to 10 minutes or less. Always protect exposed areas of skin that are not affected by psoriasis with sunscreen, and avoid extended periods in the sun.

If you prefer to avoid direct sun exposure, artificial sunlight via phototherapy may be a better option. Hand-held phototherapy wands, combs, and brushes that provide artificial sunlight have shown some success in alleviating psoriasis symptoms in studies. Check with your doctor to determine if you are a good candidate for light therapy. Sun and phototherapy may NOT be a good option for you if:

- You are pregnant.

- You have lupus or any other condition that gets worse with light exposure.
- You are at an increased risk for skin cancer.

For more information on sun therapy, see **Eczema and Red, Itchy Scalp**, page 150.

Natural Oil Therapy

Combine ¼ cup each peanut oil and olive oil and apply directly to psoriasis-affected skin areas. This mixture is believed to help heal surface skin cells and increase the scalp's elasticity. This oil therapy may be used as a pre-shampoo treatment or as a leave-in treatment, depending on your preference. If used as a pre-shampoo treatment, the hair should be covered with a plastic shower cap, and the oil should be left on the scalp overnight for best results. Alternatively, applying the oil for thirty to 45 minutes before shampooing may also relieve psoriasis symptoms in some sufferers.

Flaxseed Oil

A tablespoon of flaxseed oil taken orally each day, combined with a simple one-a-day multivitamin, may help to relieve psoriasis symptoms in some sufferers.

Herbal Tea Therapy

Herbal teas are frequently used in Chinese medicine to combat psoriasis all over the skin. Teas made of slippery elm bark, yellow saffron, or chamomile are common prescriptions. Place ¼ teaspoon of the desired herb in a cup. Pour in boiling water, and stir thoroughly until the tea is brewed. Drink a cup of tea nightly before bedtime.

NOTE: Women who are pregnant or nursing should avoid using these teas without permission from a doctor as some have been known to bring on miscarriage.

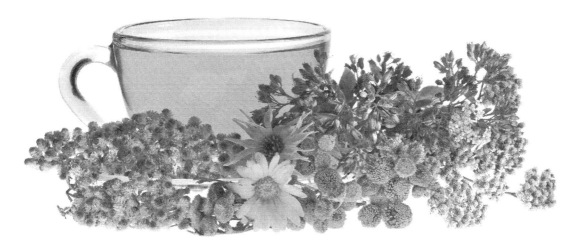

Figure 118- Herbal tea rinses may help relieve psoriasis of the scalp.

Saffron Tea Misting & Rinsing

For psoriasis of the scalp, tea misting and/or rinsing may provide some relief. Try steeping 1 or 2 teaspoons yellow saffron in 2 liters hot water in a large bowl for 15 to 20 minutes. Once steeping is complete and the water has cooled, strain the mixture and return it to the original water container. You may add the saffron-water mix to a mister bottle to spray affected areas during the day, or use it as a final scalp rinse after conditioning the hair.

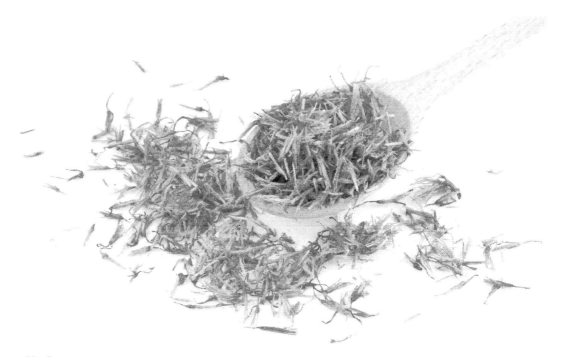

Figure 119- Try a yellow saffron tea rinse to soothe scalp psoriasis.

Ringworm

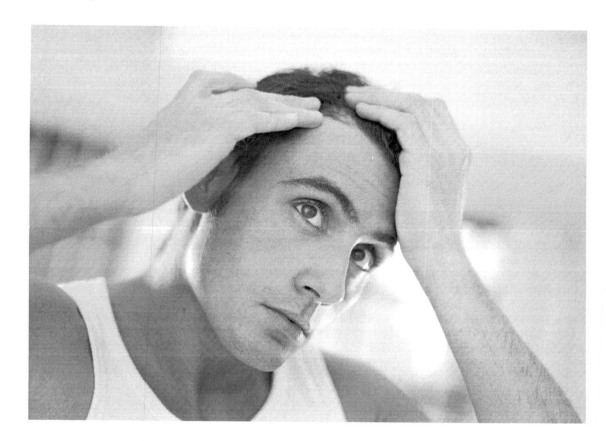

For those who have had to deal with this skin issue, ringworm can be quite embarrassing. Angry red rings may show up on faces, scalps, and literally anywhere there is vulnerable skin. To make it worse, that fiery red ring is often a death sentence for any hair in the affected region. On the scalp, ringworm (also known as *tinea capitis*) generally leaves dry, patchy, temporarily bald areas of skin. It simply causes hair in the affected region to become so brittle, that it easily breaks off. This highly contagious skin and scalp condition can easily crop up with very little warning. Luckily, ringworm is easy to treat. The tips in this section, used with your doctor's approval, may help you relieve your ringworm problem.

Signs & Symptoms

Ringworm tends to start as an itchy, red bump or dry patch of skin. As time passes, the affected area grows larger and leaves dry, itchy patches of temporary baldness. A telltale red, bumpy ring may form— and this ring feature gives ringworm its name. Interestingly, the center of the ring often appears completely clear of infection. Multiple ringworm rings are common, but in some cases there may be no rings visible at all. Signs and symptoms include:

- An excessively itchy scalp.
- Dry, scaly skin.
- A red, ringed patch made up of tiny blisters (Skin appears clear or normal inside the ring.)
- Possible hair loss contained within the area of infection.

Causes & Triggers

Contrary to popular belief, ringworm is not caused by a worm. It is caused by several types of fungi that live on the skin and hair. These fungi thrive in warm, dark, moist environments and can be passed on by direct skin-to-skin contact. Ringworm tends to be most active in the hot, summer months. Sharing or touching contaminated items such as combs, pillowcases, clothing, and infected pets (especially cats) can cause the ringworm infection to spread.

Ringworm of the scalp takes longer to develop than ringworm on other parts of the body. Scalp ringworm usually appears ten to fourteen days after contact with a contaminated source, while other forms of ringworm become visible as soon as four days after contact. When sufferers rub or scratch the infected areas and then touch other areas of the skin, secondary ringworm infections can crop up in days. Those with minor scalp injuries and poor hygiene (and those who keep their skin damp for extended periods

of time) may be at greater risk for ringworm infections.

> **When It's Time to See Your Doctor**
> Ringworm can occur on nails, hands, feet, scalp, and other skin areas and typically does not require a doctor's care. However, do see a doctor if you've developed ringworm on the scalp or if your skin begins to crack or blister.

Intervention & Preventing Relapse

Over-the-Counter Treatment

Most cases of ringworm can be cured with over-the-counter creams and ointments such as *Blue Star Ointment*, which kill off the fungi. Over-the-counter creams that contain *miconazole* or *clotrimazole* usually work as well. Iodine is also another effective treatment for ringworm. Most ringworm treatments take one to four weeks to clear up. Once the visible signs of ringworm are gone, continue your entire course of treatment as directed by your doctor.

Shampoo Therapy

In addition to antifungal creams, a dedicated shampoo regimen can help mitigate the effects of ringworm and prevent its spread. Shampoo your hair two times a week with selenium sulfide or ketoconazole-based medicated shampoo. Although these shampoos cannot stop the ringworm fungal infection, they can help slow its progress.

Tea Tree Oil

As with most skin conditions, tea tree oil is an effective remedy for ringworm infection. Perfect for antifungal conditions, tea tree oil can be diluted or used straight and applied directly to the affected area 2 or 3 times a day. First, clean the affected skin area with soap and water. Pat

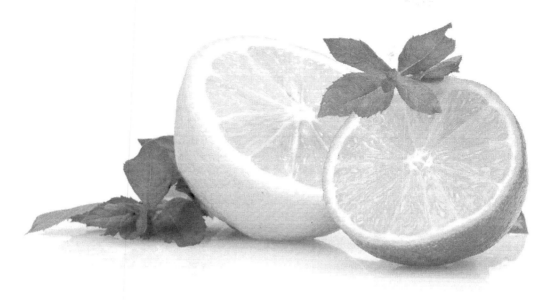

Figure 120- The power of citrus fruits like lemon or lime can help relieve ringworm in some sufferers.

the area dry, and apply 3 drops tea tree oil to a cotton swab or cotton ball. Use the cotton to dab the tea tree oil onto the ringworm, ensuring that all areas are covered with the oil. If tea tree oil is irritating to your skin at full strength, dilute 1 ½ tablespoons tea tree oil in 1 cup warm water or olive oil before dabbing the mixture onto the skin.

Apple Cider Vinegar

Apple cider vinegar is a popular remedy for ringworm. Two important acids in vinegar— malic acid and acetic acid—have antifungal and antibacterial properties that may help fight ringworm infection. Simply apply a few drops to a cotton swab or cotton ball, and dab onto the affected area twice a day.

Salt Treatment

Salt is another common home remedy for ringworm. Dab a cotton ball in water, and then dip the cotton ball in salt. Apply the cotton ball to the affected ringworm area. (Be careful, since this may sting.) Allow the salt to remain on the

area for 20 minutes and then rinse it off. Apply the salt twice daily.

Fruit Therapy

Cut a lemon or lime in half, and dip the cut side of the fruit in salt. Apply the salted lemon or lime to the infected ring for 5 to 10 minutes twice a day. If your skin is sensitive, you may skip the salt and just go with the fruit alone. Avoid scrubbing the area as this can break the skin and lead to further infection.

Castor Oil

For relief from itchy ringworm of the scalp, apply a generous amount of castor oil to the affected regions after shampooing and conditioning the hair. For additional relief, apply castor oil to the ringworm twice a day.

Disinfect Personal-Care Items

Because ringworm is quite contagious, any combs or brushes should be soaked in hot, soapy water immediately after use. Add a small capful of bleach to the water for additional protection against the fungus. Men and boys should shampoo their hair immediately after haircuts, since clippers are easy transmitters of ringworm. Keep all personal items used by someone with ringworm washed thoroughly in hot, soapy water. All clothing and towels should be dried on the hottest dryer cycle possible to prevent reinfection.

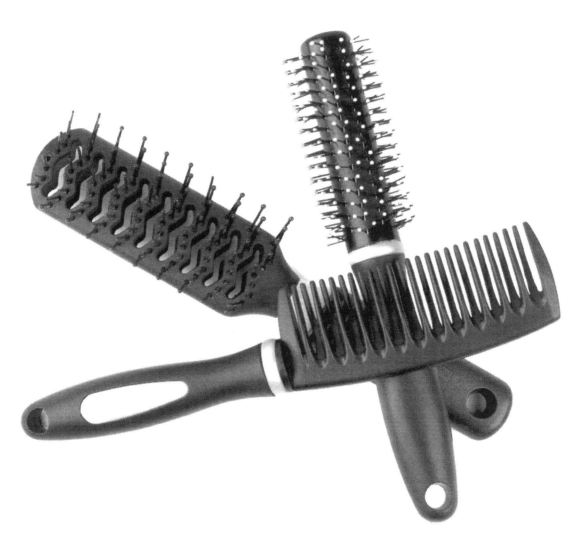

Figure 121- Personal hair care items should be disinfected to prevent the spread of ringworm.

Seborrheic Dermatitis

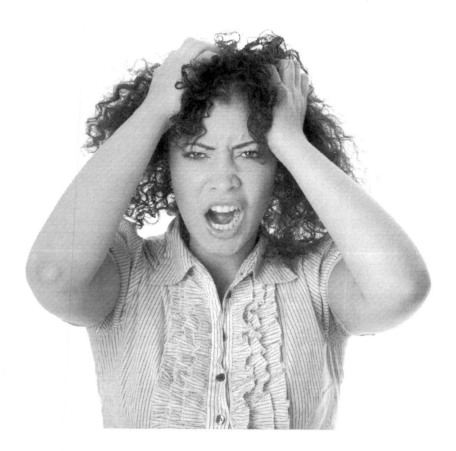

We can all imagine better things to do with our time than scratching through layers and layers of flaky, dry scalp skin. But for those who suffer from seborrheic dermatitis, batting away flakes is all in a day's work. Dry, itchy scalps with thick, flaky patches of skin are a common sight for those who suffer from seborrheic dermatitis. *And boy, are those flakes stubborn!* Seborrhea produces flakes that hug the scalp around the hairs they surround, making lifting these dreadful flakes up and out of the hair next to impossible. Nearly 30 percent of Americans have scalps blanketed in this white, scaly crust. The tips in this section, used with your dermatologist's approval, may help you relieve troublesome seborrheic dermatitis once and for all.

Signs & Symptoms

Seborrhea mimics dandruff so closely that many sufferers think they have a regular dandruff condition. When seborrheic dermatitis is present in infants and small children, the condition is known as cradle cap (see page 128).

Basic signs and symptoms of the condition include:

- Itchy, greasy, yellowish flakes on the scalp.
- Scaling and crusting made up of hard, greasy super-adherent flakes.
- Scales that appear on other areas of the body (eyebrows, around the nose, behind the ears, etc).
- Hair loss in some severe cases.

Causes & Triggers

Seborrhea tends to go through cycles of flaring up, improving, and then flaring up again. The symptoms may persist for years.

Like most scalp conditions, the exact cause of seborrhea is still a mystery. Since many cases of seborrhea respond to antifungal shampoo treatment, scientists believe that *malassezia*, the same fungus that instigates regular dandruff, may be to blame for the skin condition.

When It's Time to See Your Doctor

Seek medical attention for seborrhea if the condition worsens (dry, scaly patches spread to other parts of the body) or if there is redness, bleeding or discomfort associated with the condition.

Intervention & Preventing Relapse

Shampooing Regimen

Since some forms of seborrhea have been found to respond positively to antifungal shampoo treatment, a shampoo regimen in which zinc pyrithione-, ketoconazole-, and selenium sulfide-based shampoos are rotated on a monthly schedule may be beneficial. Because these shampoos can be hard on the hair, be sure to deep condition the hair thoroughly after each cleansing session to restore your hair's moisture balance.

The hair may need to be cleansed more regularly to remove *malassezia* overgrowth and keep the scalp in good working order.

Tea Tree Oil

Because tea tree oil has antifungal properties, applying it to affected skin may help alleviate some of the flaking caused by seborrhea and other scalp-skin conditions. Apply 3 drops tea tree oil to a cotton swab or cotton ball, and dab onto the scaly areas. If tea tree oil is too irritating on its own, simply dilute it in warm water or olive oil before applying to the skin.

Post-shampoo Rosemary Tea Rinse

A post-shampoo tea rinse may also help to alleviate troublesome seborrhea. Add 2 tablespoons *each* rosemary, witch hazel and comfrey leaves to 2 cups boiling water. Allow the tea to cool, strain out the leaves, and then add 3 to 5 drops of tea tree oil. Apply the mixture to your scalp after shampooing. After 10 minutes, rinse and condition the hair.

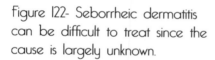

Figure 122- Seborrheic dermatitis can be difficult to treat since the cause is largely unknown.

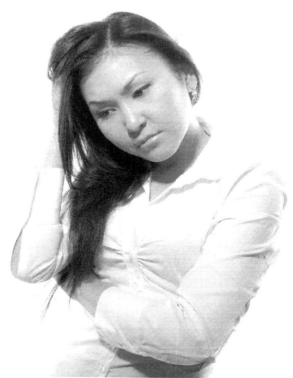

Shedding

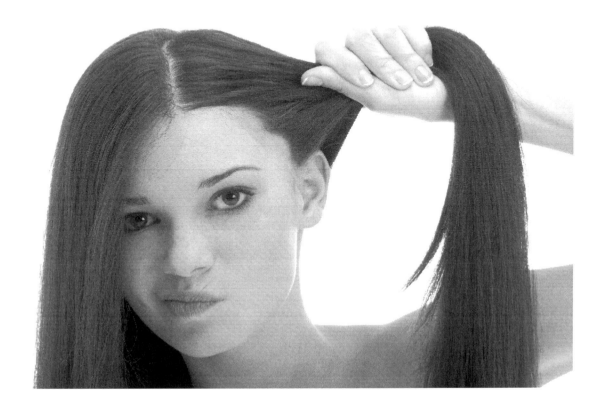

W'ere afraid we have a bit of bad news. Are you sitting down? Good. Despite what it seems, our hair follicles do not constantly produce hair. It's not a major revelation—but it's true. While follicles do spend a lot of time producing the hair we know and love, they also rest and take breaks from time to time. Our hair grows for a few years without interruption—and then stops and rests for a few weeks. When the rest period is over, the hair strand falls out and the process starts over again. This is the lifecycle of a hair strand, and the process goes on the same way for hairs all over the body. The tips in this section, with your doctor's approval, will help you understand and survive hair shedding.

Signs & Symptoms

On a typical day, most people shed fifty to one hundred hairs. But that fifty to one hundred hairs can easily feel like one thousand when you are sitting there with the equivalent of small hamster in your comb! Common signs of hair shedding include:

- Fallen hair strands with white tips on one end.
- Diffuse hair thinning throughout the scalp (in severe cases).

Although it can seem like the entire scalp is being affected by shedding, on a typical, healthy scalp, just about 10 percent of that head's hairs are ever in the rest and shedding stage. Occasionally, shedding may be restricted to a particular area of the scalp.

Shedding or Breakage?

Now, before we talk about causes and prevention, it's really important that we make a distinction *between hair shedding* and *hair breakage*. People often

confuse shedding with breakage, but there's a huge difference between the two!

Shed hairs are hairs that *naturally* fall out. These hairs always have a tiny white tip on one end

> **When It's Time to See Your Doctor**
> Shedding is a natural part of the hair-growing process, but if your rate of shedding suddenly increases beyond what is typical for you—or if you notice patchy hair loss—consult a dermatologist.

because this is the end of the hair that came from the scalp. (When your hair follicle goes into *rest mode*, it also stops producing your hair color, which is why the tip is always white or light in color). Shed hairs fall no matter how well you take care of your hair.

A broken hair, on the other hand, does not naturally fall and will have no tip to suggest

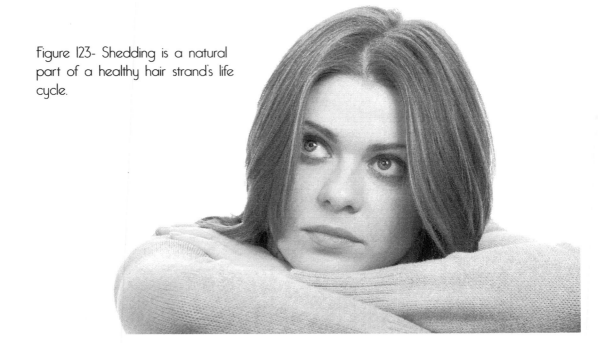

Figure 123- Shedding is a natural part of a healthy hair strand's life cycle.

that it came directly from the scalp—because it didn't. These hairs break away from healthier pieces of hair strands because of some kind of trauma to the hair. Taking better care of your hair will always reduce the occurrence of these broken hairs significantly. (See Basic Hair Breakage, page 108.)

As a rule of thumb, shed hairs tend to be longer than broken hair strands.

Causes & Triggers

Hair shedding is a natural part of living, and is really just a sign of a healthy, functioning scalp. As we get older, the number of hairs we naturally shed slowly starts to increase. But excessive shedding—very loosely and unofficially defined as "more fallen hair than you are used to seeing on a weekly or monthly basis"—can still be distressing. What causes our growing hairs to enter their resting phase and fall?

The major causes of increased hair shedding are:

- Hormonal changes associated with puberty, menstruation, pregnancy, and menopause.
- Age and heredity—runs in the family.
- Crash dieting/low-protein and low-iron diets.
- High stress.
- Severe illness, especially with high fever as a prevailing symptom.
- Certain medications (oral contraceptives and antidepressants), major surgeries, and chemotherapy.
- Low manipulation styling.
- Overworking the hair, especially with chemicals.
- Climatic/seasonal.
- Long hair (in the comb, long shed hairs may give the impression of lots more shedding than a similar number of shorter strands).

Hormonal Changes

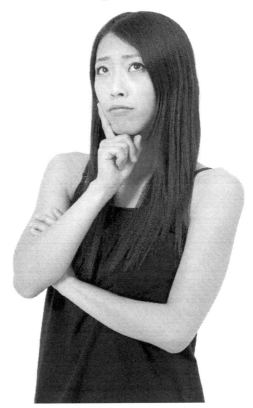

Figure 124- Hormones regulate hair shedding.

In the body, hormones control just about everything! Hair shedding is no exception to the rule. Major life events—namely puberty, menstruation, pregnancy or menopause—always tend to have an effect on the rate of hair shedding because they can really shift hormone levels.

Postpartum Shedding

Ask any woman with children, and she'll usually tell you about how amazing, vibrant, full and just plain awesome her hair was during pregnancy. This isn't just imagination at work! During pregnancy, our hormones kick into high gear with a surge of activity to prepare our bodies for making another person. This activity boost also locks the hair into its production and growing phase—and the hair grows and thrives like never before. Pregnancy hair can really be the best hair of your life!

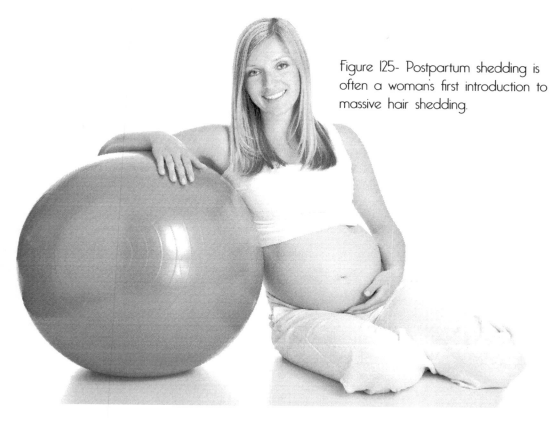

Figure 125- Postpartum shedding is often a woman's first introduction to massive hair shedding.

But you can't live the high life for too long! For many women, the arrival of baby triggers an onslaught of serious shedding and hair loss when hormone levels nosedive to return back to pre-pregnancy levels. Hairs that normally would have shed unnoticed a few at a time during the pregnancy, start to fall out together—that is, pretty much all at once!—after the pregnancy. This shedding usually occurs within the first three to six months of giving birth and may or may not occur with future pregnancies.

Contrary to popular belief, loading up with prenatal vitamins, or extending or prematurely ending nursing, won't affect the rate of shedding. Shedding will automatically begin to taper off about six months to a year after giving birth. Unfortunately, it's a "sit and wait" game.

Age & Heredity

Age and genes play a role in shedding rates. The older we are, the more likely we are to see an increase in hair shedding. As hairs shed, they aren't replaced as quickly as they were in youth. This can lead to a gradual, noticeable thinning of the scalp hair as we head into the golden years. The rate and degree of hair loss is usually genetically determined.

Nutritional Problems

Simply eating a balanced diet can work wonders for a wide range of hair issues. Nutritional deficiencies in certain vitamins and minerals, usually due to crash dieting, often lead to increased shedding rates. Diets with low protein or iron components are also particularly susceptible to increased bouts of shedding, as are high protein, high fat diets.

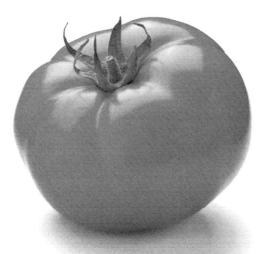

Figure 126- Eat a balanced diet to keep your shedding rate low.

Stress & Illness

Deadlines. Struggling economies. Traffic jams. Kids! High-stress living can lead to increased hair shedding for some people. Surgeries, traumatic events, and severe illness, especially conditions with high fever as a prevailing symptom, can also lead to hair loss a few weeks or months out from the actual illness. Thyroid disorders are particularly hard on the hair follicles and can trigger bouts of shedding.

Medications/Surgeries

Hair loss can be a side effect of some medications that are used to treat other health conditions. In particular, medications that are used to treat conditions such as hyperthyroid, hypothyroid, acne and even some oral contraceptives (birth control pills) can trigger bouts of shedding. Check with your doctor to see if the medication you might be taking increases hair shedding. Your doctor may be able to offer you an alternative.

Low Manipulation Styling

Believe it or not, there are times when barely handling the hair can result in what looks like inordinate amounts of shedding. Remember the 50-to-100-hairs-a-day shedding norm? If your hair is in a long-term style that does not allow you to comb it daily (weaves or braid extensions, for example), then the amount of shed hair you'll

Figure 127- Stress and illness can lead to excessive hair fall.

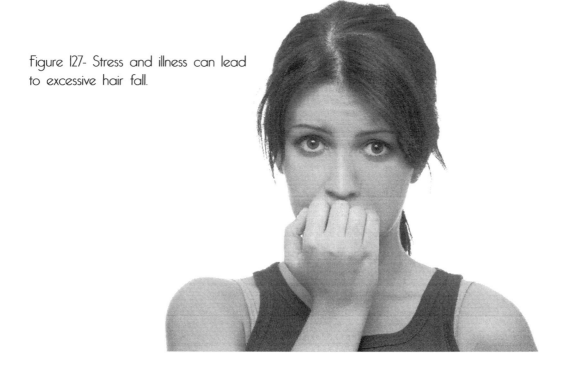

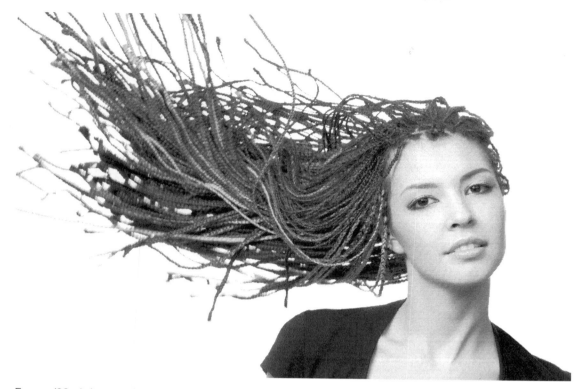

Figure 128- Wearing long-term styles such as braided extensions can increase the amount of shed hair a person sees when the style is removed. Shed hairs, trapped by the braids, accumulate over the period of time the style is worn, and then fall together at takedown.

see when you take down the style will be all of the hair you've shed throughout the total time you've worn the style. It's just that the style has retained the shed hairs instead of allowing them to fall naturally.

If, for instance, your head normally sheds 30 hair strands per day, and you've kept your style for two weeks, you could lose as many as 420 strands in one sitting (30 strands x 14 days). This amount of shedding would be completely normal—it only looks alarming because of the accumulation of hairs that would normally fall one at a time.

Overworking the Hair
Overworking the hair with chemical treatments such as relaxers, straighteners, perms, hair dyes, and bleaches can sometimes instigate shedding.

While these treatments are not intended to be applied to the scalp, it is difficult to avoid the scalp entirely. Sensitivities to these chemicals may also be a factor in shedding flare-ups.

Climate/Seasonal
Like everything else in the animal kingdom, our shedding may also respond to changes in the seasons. Some research has shown that shedding rates tend to be highest in the fall and lower in the springtime.

Intervention & Preventing Relapse
Since much of the shedding we experience is hormonal and usually turns itself around in time, shedding intervention tips tend to have limited success. If shedding really has you down, some of the tips here may be worth a try in addition to a consult with your dermatologist.

Coffee & Tea Therapy Rinses

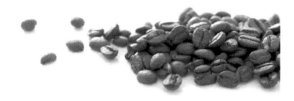

Figure 129- Caffeine applied as a rinse may help reduce hair fall.

Caffeine does more than just perk us up in the mornings. New research shows that caffeine may help block the damaging effects of some hormones on the hair follicles. Coffee and black-tea beverages are especially rich in caffeine, boasting up to 200 mg and 61 mg respectively in an 8-ounce cup. Try the following treatment rinses the next time you find yourself parting with hair:

Basic Brew
Coffee: Simply brew 2 or 3 cups of coffee as usual.

Tea: Place 2 or 3 tea bags in boiling water, and steep until dark. The amount of tea you brew will depend on how much hair you have. Simply add more tea bags (or less water) for a stronger brew.

How to Use: Whether you try coffee or tea, allow the liquids to cool before rinsing your hair with them. Pour the rinse over your hair after you've shampooed it, and gently massage it into the scalp for several minutes. Alternatively, you may put the liquid in a spray bottle and work the liquid into your most problematic areas. Allow the rinse to remain on the hair for ten minutes, and then rinse out completely. Coffee and tea rinses may have a strengthening effect on the

hair fiber, so be sure to condition the hair as needed with a moisturizing product to balance the extra strengthening.

NOTE: Coffee and black tea rinses can darken the hair over time, so if your hair is light and you'd prefer to keep it that way, you may want to avoid regular tea rinsing.

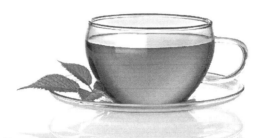

Figure 130- Black tea contains a considerable amount of caffeine. which may boost hair retention by preventing follicle damage.

Garlic Relief

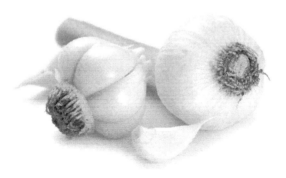

Figure 131- Garlic is an age-old remedy for hair shedding.

When your shedding has you at wit's end, try garlic. This pungent bulb has been used for years as a natural remedy for hair shedding. While the exact way that garlic helps reduce shedding is unknown, and the positive results are anecdotal at best, it can't hurt to give it a try!

Some garlic users claim to have reduced their rates of shedding by simply ingesting more raw garlic in their diets or by using garlic supplements and tablets found in many health foods stores. Others choose to add a bulb or two of crushed raw garlic to shampoos, conditioners, sprays and oil products as a direct and concentrated means of combatting the problem. To keep the garlicky smell at bay in your homemade concoctions, use the treatment as a pre-shampoo scalp oil treatment or simply mask the smell with essential oils. If you'd prefer a ready-made concoction, there are also garlic-based shampoo and conditioner products that you can purchase at your local grocer or health foods store to curb shedding. These products usually have the garlicky smell toned down considerably.

Onion Juice Therapy

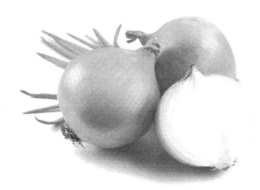

Figure 132- Onion, a close relative of garlic, is also a common treatment for shedding.

Onions are not just for the kitchen, and as a close cousin of garlic, it's no wonder the onion is on the shedding therapy list! Some interesting research on this eye-watering veggie has shown that applying onion juice to the scalp twice daily for two to three months may be effective at reducing hair shedding in some people. When you buy your onions, only select ones that have dry and crisp outer skins and show no signs of sprouting or age. Of course the jury is still out

on whether or not onion juice can really end shedding for good, but it won't hurt your wallet if it doesn't work.

Keep Styling and Manipulation Down!

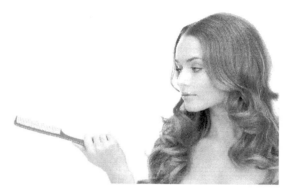

Figure 133- Keep manipulation down to a minimum when your shedding is in full swing.

If your hair is seriously shedding, the last thing you want to do is aggravate it by combing and brushing through it. While reducing your hair handling and manipulation won't actually stop hairs that are programmed to fall from falling, it will help you reduce the chances for tangling and unwanted breakage as this process does go on.

Always avoid tension bearing hairstyles such as tight ponytails, hair rollers, and extensions that can pull on your scalp since these can potentially make shedding worse.

Single-Strand Knots

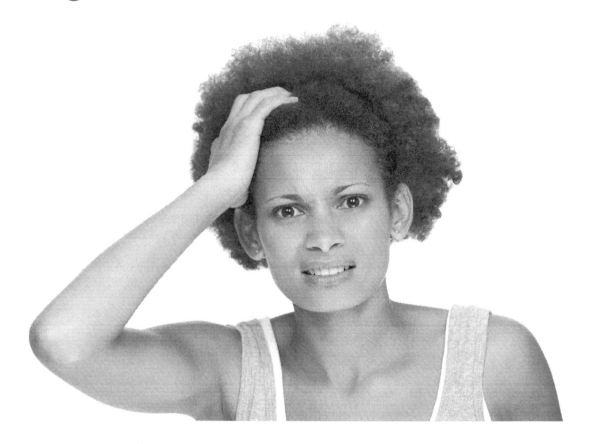

They are called by many names—*Trichonodosis*, single-strand knots (SSKs), and even fairy knots—but there is nothing magical or warm and fuzzy feeling about these microscopic tangles. Single-strand knots mean one thing for naturally curly and coily girls: Trouble. Left unchecked, these little knots can tangle your relatively healthy neighboring coils and curls into a huge, matted mess. While some knotting is normal and to be expected with natural hair—especially for the coiliest of coily hair types—don't let single-strand knots drive you over the edge! The tips in this section will help you reduce the occurrence of these annoying knots in your hair once and for all.

Signs & Symptoms

- Tiny knots resembling tiny beads on just one strand of hair. One or two knots per strand is common.
- Excessive tangling.
- Possible hair breakage.

Causes & Triggers

How do those little knots get there anyway? There are lots of theories to explain what causes single-strand knotting. These knots occur when naturally coily or curly hair bends or folds back onto itself. These knots frequently occur without much provocation or warning and are often just a natural characteristic of super-curly hair. These knots should be dealt with by snipping the strand just above the place where the knot has formed.

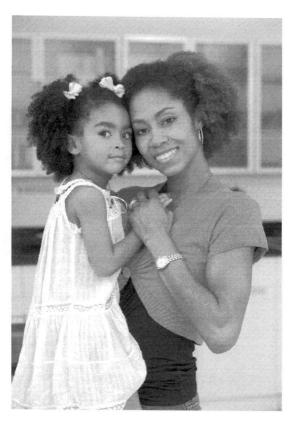

Figure 134- Single-strand knots are very common in highly-textured, kinky-coily hair.

Typical causes and triggers of knots include:

- Natural characteristic of the hair.
- Dry, poorly conditioned hair.
- Shrunken hair (usually from "wash and go" styles or hair that is not protected at night).

Intervention & Preventing Relapse

We can't prevent all knots from occurring, but we can try to keep them contained. Try these tips for drastically reducing the number of single-strand knots and other tangles in kinky-curly hair.

Keep It Hydrated!

The single best solution for single-strand knots is simply to keep the hair hydrated. Tangles are more likely to form in dried, shrunken hair than in moisturized, elastic, and stretched-out hair.

Detangle Your Hair Thoroughly

While it is undeniably time consuming, careful detangling will save you lots of hair stress and trouble down the road—especially as your coils and curls grow longer. You should always apply a softening product (moisturizer/conditioner/oil) to the hair before detangling to reduce friction. To avoid additional damage, start the detangling process using your fingers first. Always work on the hair in small, manageable sections, isolating individual hairs as you move along.

Start detangling the hair at the ends, and work up from the bottom toward the scalp. Once the hair is detangled with your fingers, you can work your way down to progressively smaller combs until you've detangled to your taste. If your hair can tolerate it, try a detangling brush like the Denman (see Frizzy Hair, page 159 for more on this brush) to polish off your detangling efforts. Continue to work slowly in sections until the entire head is thoroughly detangled.

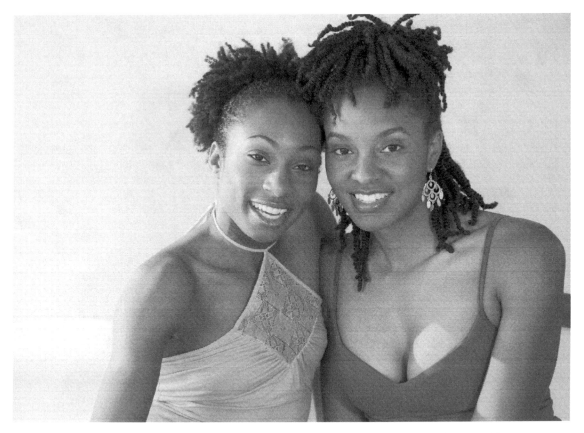

Figure 135- Keeping your hair moisturized is the best defense against single-strand knots.

Moisturize & Condition the Hair with a Vengeance

Regular attention to your hair's moisture balance will keep most single-strand knots at bay. You really want to strive for comprehensive conditioner coverage. Here's why: Typically, we condition our hair as one large unit, paying the most attention to the top and sides and barely scrunching product through the middle of the head. Add to this the fact that conditioner products on the whole aren't as spreadable on the hair as shampoos, and it's easy to leave certain parts of the hair needing a moisture boost! Be sure that you are getting conditioner to all areas of your head.

If you have a problem with knotting, moisturize or lightly mist your hair once a day to keep your curls fresh and hydrated. Follow up by sealing your hair with an oil product to prevent friction between the strands that can lead to knotting.

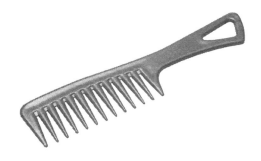

Figure 136- Working with your fingers and large-tooth combs will substantially decrease your hair's chances of knotting and tangling.

Keep It Stretched!

Shrunken hair styles are Knot Central. When curly and coily hair is allowed to shrink into its tightest (default) configuration, the hair is primed for knotting! Curls and coils love to intermingle with their neighbors and even coil back onto themselves. Afros, puffs, and wash-n-go curls are the number-one single-strand-knot culprits—especially if the styles are worn for several consecutive days. Try stretching out your hair as much as possible with twists, braids, and fluffed-out variations of these styles.

At night, protect your hair by plaiting or twisting it to lengthen the curls and coils. Cover the hair with a satin scarf or bonnet to reduce friction between your hair and bedding.

Wear It Shorter

If all else fails, consider wearing your hair at a shorter length (less than 3 to 4 inches) to reduce the occurrence of single-strand knots and tangling. Shorter hair is much easier to work with and is less likely to knot on itself than lengthier tresses.

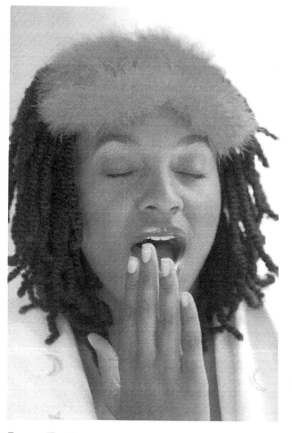

Figure 137- Keep your hair stretched and protected at night.

Sluggish Hair Growth

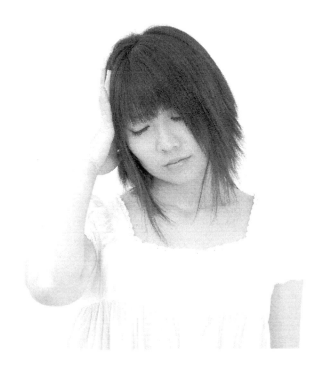

Maybe you've just gotten the worst haircut of your life, or you simply want your shorter hair to fit into that snazzy updo for your wedding or special occasion a few months away—either way you are having the hair-growing blues. But, before you reach for the next Megagrowth Super Hair Vitamin or some other magical oil or cream, realize that these products rarely deliver on their promises. Why? Because they cannot get around the inconvenient little fact that hair growth is a process that is regulated by hormone activity. Unless products work on the hormonal level, they can't work to grow hair. (See Hair Loss & Thinning, page 175, to learn about prescription products that CAN grow hair). The tips in this section will help you get back on the road to healthy hair growing once and for all.

Signs & Symptoms

Barring medical issues, the average hair on your scalp grows about 1/2 inch per month. This monthly hair allotment can be affected by things like the time of year, your personal hair practices, diet, age, and genetics. If your hair is growing pretty close to the 1/2 inch per month rate, you are not suffering from sluggish growth—you're suffering from overly high expectations!

You may have a hair-growing problem if:

- Hair growth is less than ½ to ¼ inch per month.
- There is no length accumulation over a period of several months.

Causes & Triggers

Sluggish hair growth can really be two distinct problems. The first type of hair growth problem comes from health-related issues that affect hair emergence at the scalp level; the second (and perhaps most likely) type of problem is simply poor length retention at the ends of the hair. These issues can crop up individually or may develop together.

When Health Affects Hair Growth

Keeping your body healthy by eating a well-balanced diet, drinking lots of water, and getting adequate exercise and sufficient rest will usually ensure that you experience good hair growth results month to month. But sometimes, even this is not enough. When slow hair growth is related to a health problem, the rate of hair emergence from the scalp is affected. These types of growth problems are harder to deal with because they can creep up on us out of nowhere, and they often require medical intervention to get under control.

If your hair is suffering, despite a seemingly great bill of health, have your hormone levels checked.

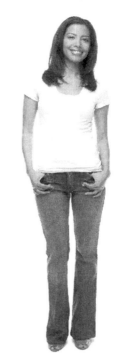

Figure 138- Many times, we are responsible for our own sluggish hair growth.

Our hormones directly influence hair growth because they regulate follicle activity. Not only do they tell our cells when to divide and when to rest, they even tell our hair follicles when to drop hair! Low estrogen levels have long been linked to sluggish growth, premature hair thinning, and hair loss, particularly during menopause.

Slow growing hair may also be a sign that your hair follicles' active growing phase is short. (All hair grows for a designated period, usually two to ten years, and then naturally sheds). If your active growing phase is short (closer to 2 years), you may have trouble reaching really long lengths such as the waist and beyond.

Our hair's growth rate and active growing periods also decrease naturally with age. So, if you are middle-aged and notice that your hair is not growing as quickly as it used to—this may be completely normal.

When YOU are Affecting Hair Growth

When slow hair growth is not related to a health or medical problem, it is usually just a hair-retention problem. Put simply—we just aren't keeping what we're growing for a variety of reasons! Ask anyone with dark hair who has bleached it: "Roots" are a constant problem because hair is always growing! Unlike health-related sluggish growth, this type of "slow hair growth" must be addressed from the ends of the hair— not the scalp. Fortunately, it is also much easier to treat!

Intervention & Preventing Relapse

While there is very little you can do to sprout hair overnight, here are a few tips that will help you ensure that the hair you do grow has the best chance of survival.

Revamp Your Diet!

Diets that are not up to snuff can seriously affect your hair. Hair follicles, skin, and nails are last on the list to receive nutrition from the body, so if your diet is marginal, your hair growth will

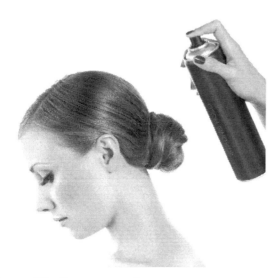

Figure 139- Protective styling can encourage faster length accumulation since hair is protected from damage.

be as well. Also remember that dietary changes from the inside do not manifest on the outside overnight . . . or even within a month or two. You'll need at least three consistent months of optimal nutrition to notice improvement. Although it is very popular to cut carbs or to cut proteins, grains, or whatever is recommended for cutting in this year's trendy diet craze-avoid restrictive-food-group dieting as much as possible. Balanced, healthy eating is critical for hair growth. If your diet needs help, consider taking a basic multivitamin to cover your weak areas.

Essential Oils

Oils such as peppermint, rosemary, and thyme work wonderfully to stimulate and encourage healthy blood flow to the hair follicles. Whether this stimulation truly encourages hair growth has yet to be proven— but if you've got to try something try the essential oil massage recipe in *Hair Loss & Thinning*, p. 181.

Protect Your Hair

Protective styling is more than just wearing a certain hair style; it is an entire way of handling and thinking about your hair. The less we handle and mess with our hair, the better it will look and the longer it will grow. If you are having an issue with slow growth—especially slow growth that is brought on by poor retention—consider weaning your hair from heat abuse or chemical treatments, or at least extending the timeframe between these services. Wear your hair up and out of the way more often, and you'll keep your hair from being worn out before its time. Handle your hair with care when shampooing, conditioning, and styling. Take time to work on your hair. You're worth it!

Give It Time

If you are growing out a particularly short cut—a pixie or cropped cut, for instance—give your

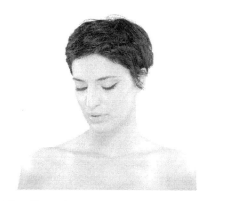

Figure 140- Short hair is naturally protective.

hair three to four months of dedicated growing time before you have your stylist even up the hair. In another three to four months, have him/her even your hair up again. If your hair is of the

faster-growing variety, you will have a short bob that is picking up length in no time.

Honestly, if you haven't noticed already, the hair-growing process is like watching paint dry on the wall! Keep fighting the good fight, and stay encouraged. Performing just these small, beneficial steps consistently over time will produce great results!

Cheat a Little!

When all else fails, and you've got to achieve a certain style on short notice, try weaving in a bit of hair to help you achieve your style of choice. If you continue to take care of your hair while you wear your extensions, it will reach your desired length in no time.

Figure 141- Healthy, lengthy hair is not beyond your reach.

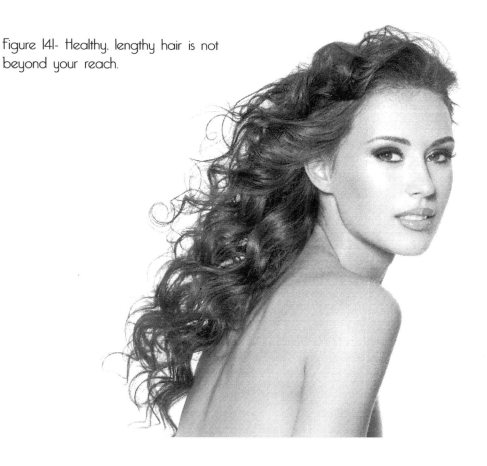

Split Ends

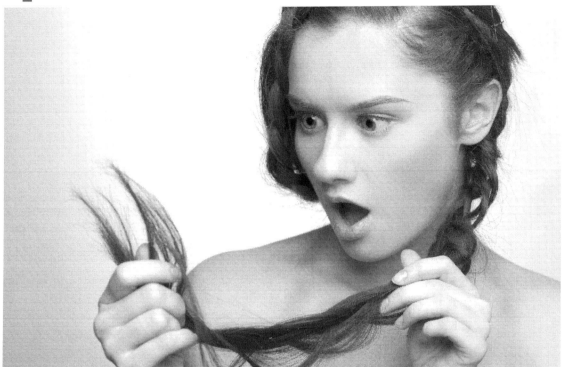

No matter how well you care for your hair, you will—at some point or another—come face to face with a split end. Split ends happen to everyone, and the longer your hair grows, the more they'll become an intimate part of your life. Split ends are caused by many types of hair trauma but typically are the result of a low moisture balance within the hair strand. When hair is allowed to remain dry, brittle, and undermoisturized for extended periods of time, the cuticle begins to crack and unravel, exposing the cortex of the hair and creating a split end.

Signs & Symptoms

- Excessive tangling near the ends of the hair.
- Dry, dull, lackluster hair—particularly near the ends.
- Split strands and breakage.
- Uneven hair.

Causes & Triggers

Split ends can crop up at any time, even in hair that is pretty well maintained. Damage from split ends often comes from:

- Excessive heat use.
- Poorly made styling tools.

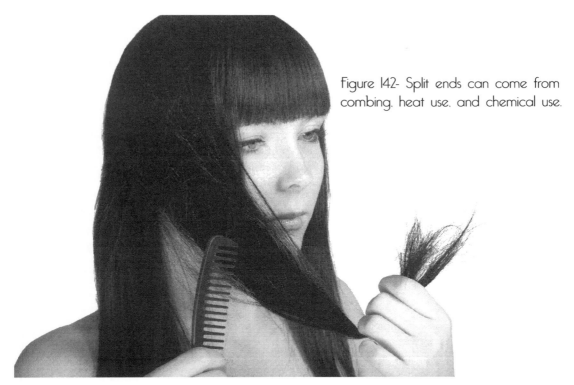

Figure 142- Split ends can come from combing, heat use, and chemical use.

- Chemical treatments.
- Weather/environment.

Heat Use

Because heat rapidly depletes the moisture balance within the hair shaft, heat use is perhaps the number-one contributor to split ends on otherwise healthy hair. Heat use can damage a perfectly healthy strand of hair in just seconds. Frequent use of heat-styling tools will increase your chances of sustaining cuticle damage and splitting ends.

Styling tools

Before your hair strand actually splits, its outer layer gets chipped, roughed up and damaged first. Poorly made styling tools such as serrated combs, hard plastic-bristle brushes, ponytail holders with metal crimps, and sharp hairpins all put the hair in danger of splitting at any point along the shaft.

But, interestingly, an often overlooked cause of troublesome split ends among styling tools is your pair of hair shears. Trimming your hair with any old pair of scissors will damage freshly cut ends before they even have a chance! Dull shears will just push your hair around in the blades before they make a fairly random (and extremely damaging) cut—not a good look!

Go for professional shears that are specifically designed for trimming the hair. These shears tend to have a sharper, more precise cutting surface and last a great deal longer than regular scissors.

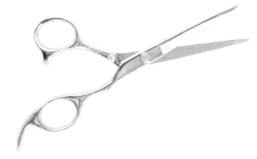

Figure 143- Bad scissors are a common cause of split ends on otherwise healthy hair.

Chemical Treatments

Chemical relaxing and permanent hair coloring degrade the cuticle in order to perform their specific functions. When the cuticle is broken down, weakened, and compromised, the hair will fracture and split. Chemical treatments are a major cause of splits that occur high up on the hair shaft rather than at the very ends.

Harsh Shampoos

Shampoos that are too harsh will sap the hair of its precious moisture content. Frequent usage of these cuticle-stripping shampoos may cause the hair to become more vulnerable to splitting over time. Always use gentle shampoo formulations, preferably sulfate-free lines.

The Elements (Sun, Wind, Cold, Arid Air)

The sun is yet another moisture-eliminating element. Its oxidative effects on the hair can make splitting problems worse. Combine the sun with other elements such as wind and cold, and the hair does not stand a chance.

Moisturizing and sealing the hair is extremely important for protecting it against damage from the elements, especially if you live in an extreme climate.

Intervention & Preventing Relapse
Stay on Top of Deep Conditioning

The best way to cure split ends is by preventing them in the first place. Work with sulfate-free cleansers whenever possible and commit to a dedicated deep conditioning regimen to strengthen the hair. Although split ends cannot really be repaired, glued back together, or eliminated by conditioning once they happen, conditioning will always improve the look of your hair.

Some protein reconstructors and serums will buy you time by temporarily sealing the ends of the hair shaft back together, but this "glue effect" is lost once the hair is exposed to water through shampooing. Ultimately, your splitting ends will need to be trimmed away.

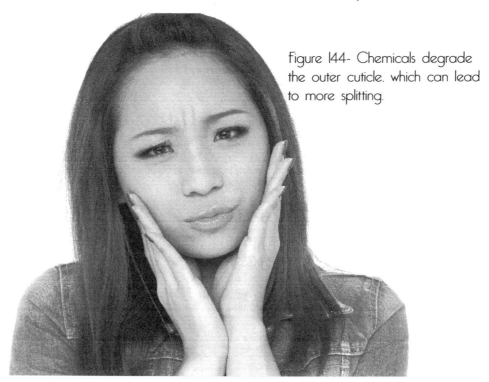

Figure 144- Chemicals degrade the outer cuticle, which can lead to more splitting.

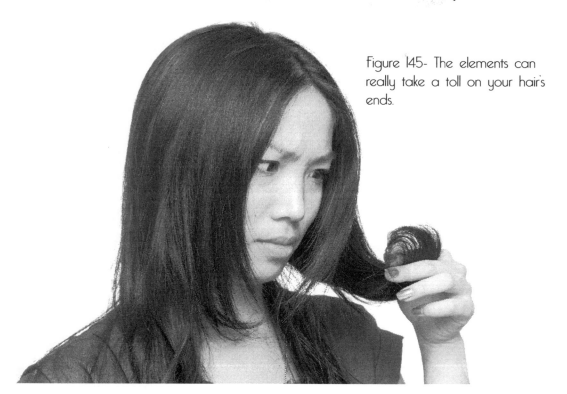

Figure 145- The elements can really take a toll on your hair's ends.

Trim the Split Ends

Most people hate having their hair trimmed—and for good reason. One trip to the salon can set you back several months in hair growth if you haven't been taking the best care of your hair. But two special types of do-it-yourself trims have gained popularity in recent years. While they aren't as precise as an all-over salon cut, they may be able to spare you some hair.

Search & Destroy Trims

The *search-and-destroy trim*, a term coined in online hair forums, is a trim that only targets individual hairs with split ends. To perform a search-and-destroy trim, simply hold up a section of hair ends to the light, and scan the tips for splitting or weak-looking strands. If you spot a splitting hair, simply trim that single hair just above its split portion. These trims are great because they do not cut healthy hairs and are undetectable. Search-and-destroy trims may be done every four weeks (or as often as needed) to keep split ends under control.

Dusting Trims

A second type of hair-saving trim is the *dusting* trim. Dusting is a "micro-trim" in which just the very tips of a hair section are removed. These trims are mainly used as preventive maintenance against split ends. Unlike search-and-destroy trims, which identify and snip individual splits only, the dusting process may remove the ends of some healthy hairs. The hair that collects on the floor after a dusting, however, is so fine and minimal that it resembles dust—hence the name. Very little hair is lost!

Because these trims are less invasive than standard trims (in which several inches of length may be cut in one sitting), they are great for maintaining the hair in between visits to a stylist.

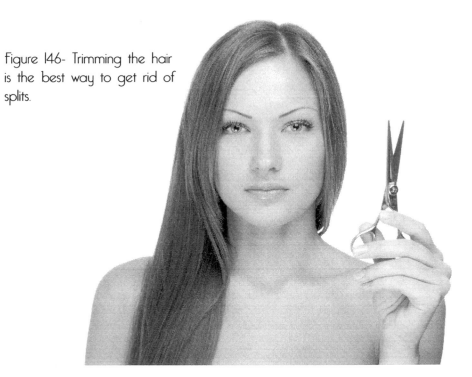

Figure 146- Trimming the hair is the best way to get rid of splits.

Decrease Hair Manipulation

Hair that is frequently manipulated and styled is vulnerable to splitting. Use protective measures when combing, brushing, and styling your hair to reduce split ends.

One of the most damaging things we do to our hair happens just after we've shampooed and conditioned it—towel drying! Although it seems innocent enough, scrunching and rubbing through our hair with fluffy terry-cloth towels can really take a toll on our tresses. To avoid damage when drying your wet hair, keep your hair hanging downward in its natural position and gently squeeze out water with your hands in a milking fashion (See Figure 117). Pat the hair dry using a microfiber towel or T-shirt to release any excess water from the hair. For more on protective styling, see page 92.

Low-pH Cuticle-Flattening Rinses

Rinsing the hair periodically with an acidic rinse (see Special Hair Conditioning & Restoration Treatments, page 250) will help to keep the cuticles flat and intact, staving off split ends. Ideally, such rinses should be done every two to three weeks as preventive maintenance against splitting and to combat problems with hair porosity. Rinsing the hair in very cool water following a wash will also help to mechanically close down the cuticle layers, preventing splits from forming.

Moisturizing & Sealing

Moisturizing and sealing the hair will help it resist splitting and hair breakage. This product-layering technique provides the cuticle with a protective barrier against the sun and other types of environmental damage that can lead to splitting. Those with fine or oily hair can find similar protection using a light leave-in spray or lotion to protect the hair against splitting as needed. Review *Hair Care Rehab: Steps 3 and 4* (pages, 85-91) for more information.

Sun & Surf Damage

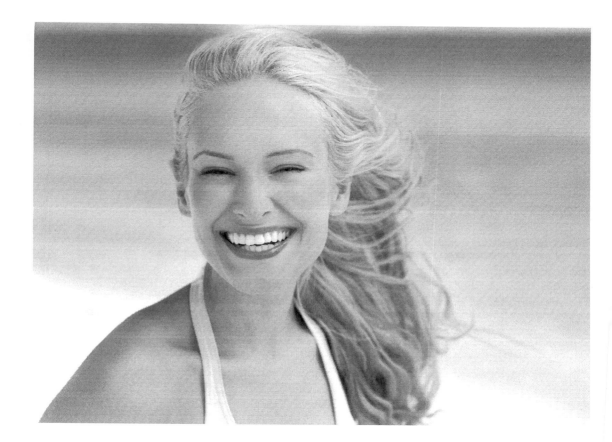

Most of us are aware of what the blazing summer sun can do to our delicate skin, but few people realize the damage our hair faces as well. The summer sun can seriously wreck and ravage our hair—especially if we combine sun and surf. Add those hot summer rays to the ocean's salty sea spray, and we're in for some serious hair repair work! Although sun-damaged hair can never be fully repaired to its original status, the tips in this section will help you improve the appearance of your hair and help prevent damage from the summer elements.

Signs & Symptoms

- Excessive hair dryness.
- Swollen, puffy hair.
- Dull, lackluster hair.
- Rampant hair breakage.

Causes & Triggers

The major causes of sun and surf damage are:

- Unprotected exposure to sun and surf.

Most hair damage comes from the combined effect of sun and surf. Why? The sun's warm rays may feel great on the skin, but it breaks down the natural protein in our hair, making our strands much more porous and dry. Ocean water looks serene and harmless, but damage from the salts found naturally in the surf can scratch and abrade the cuticle, leading to parched, dry tresses.

Wet hair and sun do not mix. Sun damage is most potent when the hair is damp. Wet hair is equivalent to focusing the sun's rays on the hair with a magnifying glass, amplifying the effects of sun damage on our hair's cuticles. The damage can be especially hard on the hair on those beach days when the hair is wet, dried in the sun, and then wet again repetitively. Can we say, *hair torture?*

Intervention & Preventing Relapse

Stay on Top of Deep Conditioning

As you may have noticed, deep conditioning the hair is important for remedying a wide variety of hair problems—and sun and surf damage is certainly no exception. Hair that is regularly deep conditioned with moisture-rich conditioning products always fares better when exposed to both sun and surf.

Create a Barrier

You may have also noticed that some products, namely conditioners and moisturizers, may come

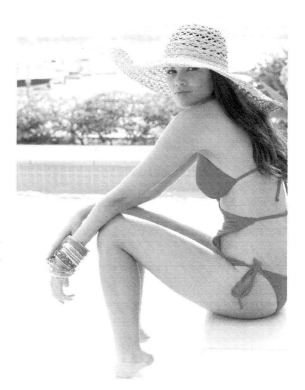

Figure 147- Wear a hat to protect your hair from the harsh, summer rays.

with sunscreens already built into the formula. Although the inclusion of sunscreens in hair products has become all the rage, the jury is still out on whether these products are actually any more effective at preventing sun damage—especially when they are included in rinse-out products. For best results, look for leave-in type products that contain sunscreens—or, simply add a bit of your regular sunscreen to your hair products to protect your hair from the harsh glare of the sun. Any barrier to the sun is better than no barrier.

Shield your hair from sun and surf damage by covering your hair with a hat or scarf when you anticipate long days in the summer sun. Wear protective hair styles such as buns or simple braids that reduce the exposure of delicate ends.

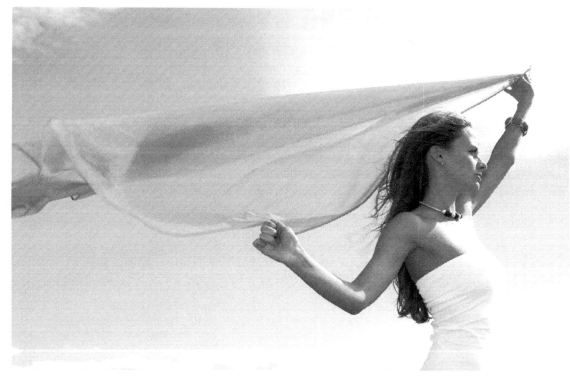

Figure 148- Scarves can protect the hair from sun and wind.

Replace Lost Protein

After long sun exposures, you'll always want to reinforce your hair with protein conditioning. Because the sun's UV rays cause most of their damage by destroying the hair's keratin proteins, protein replacement is critical to the recovery process. Apply a protein-reconstructing formula to freshly shampooed hair, and follow with a moisturizing conditioner to aid in detangling, if needed. With these new temporary proteins in place following "reconstruction," sun-damaged hair is able to hold moisture more easily.

Rinse Salty Hair ASAP

Although some people experience amazingly soft hair after a day at sea (yes, sea water can have a softening effect), salt is still quite damaging to the hair. To avoid the abrasive effects of salt, always rinse salt from the hair immediately with fresh, clean water. Never allow saltwater to dry on your strands. Conditioning your hair with moisture will make it soft, supple, and pliable again. Treat your hair to a thorough cleansing and deep conditioning with a moisture-rich shampoo and conditioner formula.

Keep Hair Dry to Reduce Sun Damage

When water, fun and sun are combined, the effect is especially hard on our delicate tresses. If you must venture out with wet hair, simply coat your exposed hair in a light instant conditioner or moisturizer prior to stepping out. Your best bet of course is to keep the hair dry whenever possible by protecting it with a swim cap, scarf, or hat.

Fake It!

If you love and must have that loose, wavy just-back-from-the-beach look—get it with less damage by using a sea-salt spray product

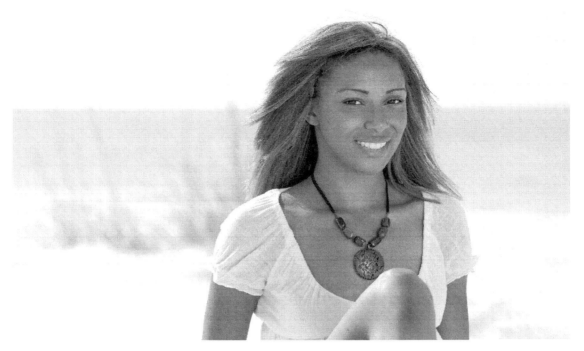

Figure 149- Color-treated hair is especially vulnerable to damage from the elements.

like Bumble and Bumble Surf Spray or Paul Mitchell Awapuhi Wild Ginger Texturizing Sea Spray (about $13-$20 on Amazon.com). These products contain other conditioning agents to protect your hair. If these sprays are pricier than you'd like, try making your very own Ocean Spray (see Special Hair Conditioning & Restoration Treatments, page 257). Salt can be drying, so always use these types of products in moderation. If dryness is a problem, apply a light leave-in conditioner to the hair before misting with your sea salt spray.

Tangly Hair

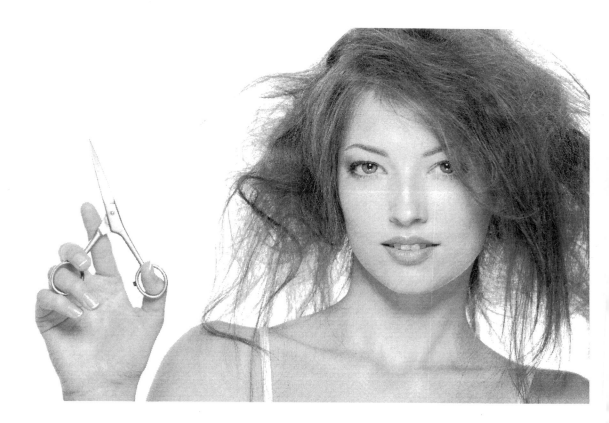

While the deliberately disheveled, bedhead look is the hot new in thing in Hollywood, it's not so chic when the tangles are not intentional! While tangles are often associated with childhood, they can follow us into the adult years as well. Tangled locks are not exclusive to any particular hair type, but they can be especially common for those with naturally curly or kinky-curly hair. If your tangled hair brings you to tears, the tips in this section will help you deal with tangles and address them before you are forced to reach for a pair of scissors.

Signs & Symptoms

- Dry, matted hair.
- Swollen, puffy hair.
- Dull, lackluster hair.

Causes & Triggers

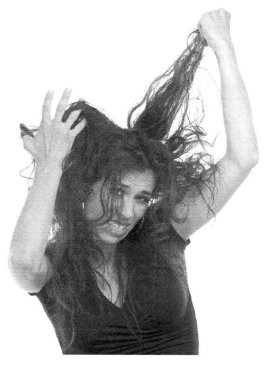

Figure 150- Tangles and snags can affect everyone.

Whenever the smooth outer surface of the hair fiber is changed, stripped or damaged—our chances for tangling increase. Tangles are caused when hair fibers mix, mingle, and mat with other hair fibers in a haphazard way. They can also be caused by static from rubbing against other materials such as bedding and clothing. Major causes of tangles and snags are:

- Natural hair shape/type.
- Hard water use.
- Chemical-processing and styling choices.

Hair Shape/Type

Our hair's length and shape can naturally lead to tangles. Uneven hair is prone to tangling because the lengths are not uniform and can easily catch on one another. Long hair is prone to tangling due to its length, and wavy, curly, and coily tresses are susceptible to tangling because of the density and shape of the hair fibers. Cutting uneven or long hair will quickly reduce tangles. Straightening or stretching out wavy, curly or kinky-curly hair will also reduce the number of tangles; however, using heat or chemical processes to achieve the change always weakens the hair.

Water Problems

Did you know that your water can lead to tangly, matted hair? Hard water is notorious for tangling the hair because it leaves dulling mineral deposits on the hair. These deposits create a rough, uneven surface on the hair fiber, leaving it primed for tangles. Harsh clarifying shampoos can also encourage tangling by stripping the hair of the natural oils that allow the hairs to move freely past one another.

Styling Choices

Our styling habits can increase our hair's tendency to tangle. Hair that has been chemically processed in any way is susceptible to tangling because the outside of the hair shaft is no longer as smooth or flat as it was before the treatment. Teasing, backcombing, blow drying and too frequent brushing of the hair can also lead to the same outcome. The swollen, chipped, and lifted cuticles these practices create are more likely to intermingle with and catch onto neighboring hair fibers, which leads to more matting and tangling.

While too much handling can certainly lead to tangling, wearing hairstyles that do not need to be combed every day can also lead to tangling. Styles that are kept beyond a week are the main

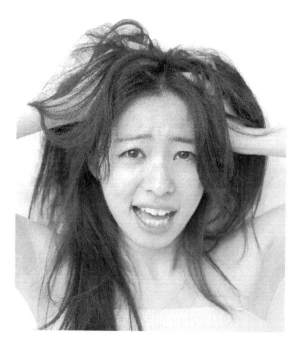

Figure 151- Tangly hair can be caused by water problems.

culprits. Hairs that would have naturally fallen as daily shed hairs aren't able to fall until the style is released. This loss of hair is natural, but these hairs—retained well past their expiry date by a protective style—can mix and mingle with hair that isn't ready to fall quite yet. This intermingling of hairs on the way out with hairs that are intact can lead to tangling issues.

Intervention & Preventing Relapse

Preventing tangles is a whole lot easier than fixing them! Try these tangle-free intervention steps to help keep your hair under control and securely on your head!

Keep a Regular Detangling Routine

Strive to detangle the hair on a regular basis. Attack tangles before they can grow into massive problems. Remember, a tangling situation will only grow worse as time passes. If you notice any hair tangling or matting, address it immediately.

Here are some simple detangling tips that you can use to cut down on tangles and snags:

1. Plasticize your hair with a mist of water, a light detangling leave-in conditioner, moisturizer, or oil before starting the detangling process. The lubricating product will help smooth the hair and loosen your tangles.

2. Always begin detangling the hair with the fingers and then move to a large-tooth comb to refine the detangling. You may then use progressively smaller combs (or a paddle brush if your hair is long) as the hair becomes easier to work through if you desire.

3. As you detangle, be sure to work the hair slowly in sections, starting at the very ends of the hair. Attempting to detangle large amounts of hair all at once can be frustrating and even damaging to the hair. If you meet a tangle in the section you're working on, reverse-engineer it (i.e., determine how the tangle is configured, and work backward to disentangle it).

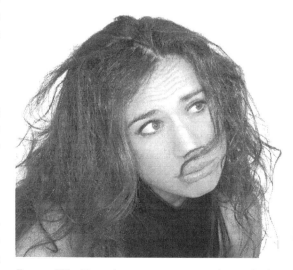

Figure 152- Hair that is not trimmed regularly to maintain a uniform length is prone to tangling between the layers.

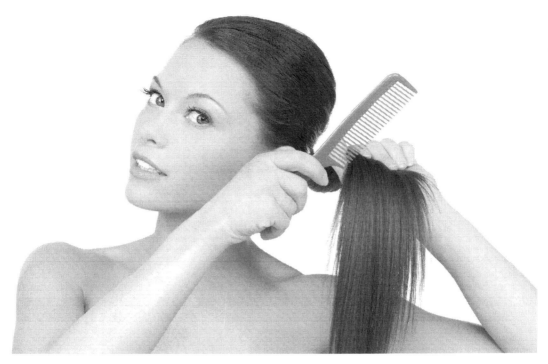

Figure 153- Regular detangling is essential to prevent bigger tangles from forming.

4. If your hair is naturally prone to tangling, always follow your shampoo with a conditioner product. Keep your hair fibers facing downward when you wash to avoid creating tangles.

5. Have a really bad tangle? Load the tangled hair up with conditioner or oil and slowly attempt to free individual or very small pieces of hair until the tangle is no more. In extreme cases, the tangle may need to be carefully snipped out.

Tangle-Free Night Care

Do you wake up with tangled, knotted hair each morning? To reduce hair tangling and matting from tossing and turning, carefully detangle and gather the hair into a loose bun, braid, or ponytail before bed. Additionally, you can try covering the hair with a satin bonnet or satin scarf nightly to keep your hair in place. If bonnets and scarves are not for you, try switching from cotton to satin pillowcases— they'll further reduce your chances for hair tangling at night.

Tangle-Free Drying

Many people hop out of the shower and briskly scrunch a towel through their hair to dry it. Unfortunately, this drying method can roughen up the cuticles and lead to unnecessary tangling. Instead, apply a detangling leave-in conditioner, and if your hair is straight (or you plan to wear it straight), gently squeeze the hair downward in a milking fashion to get rid of excess water. If your hair is wavy or curly, you'll want to cup the ends of the hair in your palm and squeeze them gently back up toward the scalp to bring out some curls.

When air drying the hair, air dry with control! Avoid allowing the hair to dry without coating

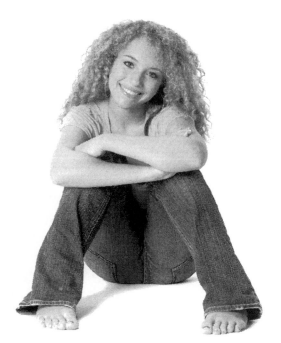

Figure 154- Always air dry your hair with control. Use finishing products to define your style.

freeform kinky-curly hairstyles look even better days out from the original set—they can become a tangling nightmare on wash day. Loose styles such as afros, twist-outs, and braid-outs are common tangling culprits. To keep tangles to a minimum, avoid wearing kinky-curly hair that is longer than three to four inches in length out for more than two to four days at a time.

Some braids and weave styles can be worn for several months at a time without combing. This is great for protecting the hair from regular styling, but it can also mean extra tangles later on. The key to avoiding tangling and matting from long-term-wear styles is to simply avoid wearing them for longer than eight to twelve weeks at a time. If your hair is prone to tangling, four to

it with a leave-in conditioner or moisturizing product. If your hair is wavy or curly, it's best to either set your damp hair with careful, organized scrunching to bring out the wave or curl pattern or to smooth the hair into a sleek shape to keep the hair from roughening or frizzing. If your hair is kinky-curly, avoid allowing the hair to shrink back onto itself during the drying process. Stretch the hair out with twists or braids so that it dries in a lengthened state.

Avoid Teasing & Backcombing Your Hair
This is a no-brainer! By definition, these processes rely on tangling the hair to bring volume and height to flat hair. Unfortunately, this process is extremely damaging to the hair and can result in some serious unintentional tangling.

Tangles & Working with Textured Hairstyles
One benefit of kinky-curly hair is that it can often accommodate hairstyles that can be worn for many days without a redo. While some

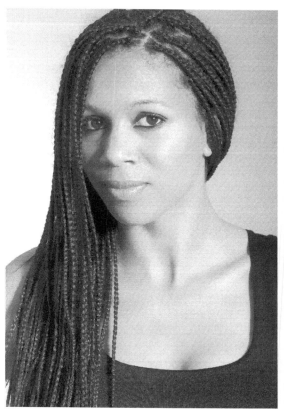

Figure 155- Textured hair types are especially prone to tangling. Contained styles keep the tangles to a minimum.

eight weeks may be the longest your hair can go in these confined styles.

The Toughest Tangle in Hair Care

The infamous "gum-stuck-in-hair" problem often leads to the mother of all tangles! Over the years, many remedies have been proposed to get gum out of hair. Slathering the gummy knot with peanut butter is a common solution. Peanut butter, though, doesn't have any special powers; it's merely the oiliness of peanut butter that makes it such an excellent gum remover.

In addition to peanut butter, many other oily household products can get gum out of hair. Alternatives to peanut butter include petroleum jelly, hair grease, vegetable oil, olive oil, mayonnaise, hair serum, and even hair mousse. Simply section the unaffected hair into a ponytail so that you can zoom in on the gummy tangle. Drench the tangled section with your oily product of choice, and work it into the gum and surrounding tangle for a minute or so. Then, carefully comb out the gum. Some have tried using toothpaste, alcohol, and even mouthwash with success, but you want to steer clear of anything that will dry out your hair needlessly.

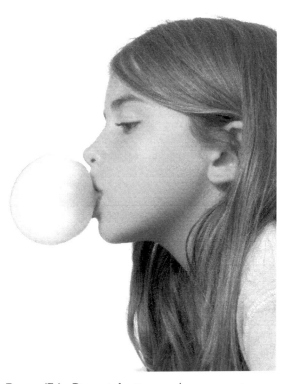

Figure 156- Peanut butter and mayonnaise are two of the many household products often used for gum removal.

Thinning Hair Edges

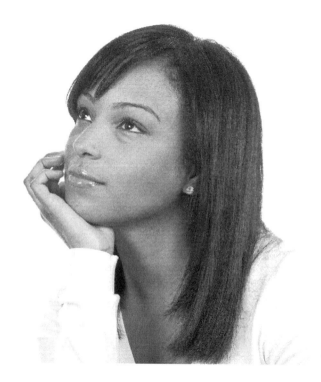

Are your edges and hairline moving farther and farther back? Do you notice more scalp in areas where hair once flourished? Thinning hair around the edges of the hairline can be brought on by a number of factors. Post-pregnancy hormone dives, birth-control methods, and simply sleeping more on one side can cause hair to thin out. Although hair thinning around the perimeter of the head can occur with almost any hair type, this type of hair damage is most common among those with highly textured hair types. This section will show you simple ways to combat a thinning head of hair around the frontal hairline, sides, and the nape of the neck.

Signs & Symptoms

- Fine, sparse hair around the hairline or nape.
- Halo-effect around the face and back hairline, where short hairs stick out from the main style.
- Excessive hair thinning and breakage near the hairline or nape.

Causes & Triggers

Hair loss anywhere can be distressing. The major causes of hair thinning around the frontal hair line, edges, and nape area are:

- Hair tension from styling choices.
- Harsh facial cleansers.
- Genetics.
- Poor diet.
- Other physical damage and heat abuse.
- Chemical overprocessing.

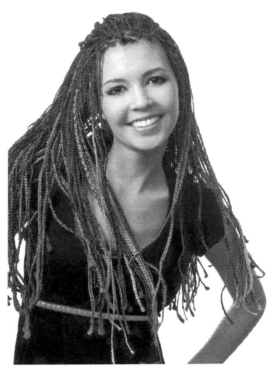

Figure 157- Braids are notorious for creating tension along the delicate hairline.

Hair Tension/Traction

The most common cause of hair thinning along the hairline is from the styling choices we make. The tension required to get certain hairstyles to lie flat or remain taut (especially when the hair type is naturally engineered to stand away from the head) can place major stress on the hair follicles—and the affected hairs may eventually fall out.

Ponytail tension is the leading cause of hairline thinning and breakage from basic styling. You can easily see this type of high-tension hair loss among athletes (i.e. dancers, gymnasts, and others) who frequently smooth their hair back into tight, controlled styles. Hats, sports sweatbands, head bands, hair extensions, weaves, and wigs and their ill-fitting linings may also rub the hairline and lead to breakage in all hair types. High-tension roller setting can also stress the hair along the frontal hairline in nearly every hair type.

Facial Cleansers

Still another possible cause of thinning along the frontal hairline for all hair types is harsh facial cleansers. Many times, the hair that frames our face is washed daily with our favorite cleanser or acne product. These cleansers are often very hard on our delicate hairlines and may dry out the hair, making it brittle and breakage-prone. If you are having hairline issues, evaluate this area of your routine.

Genetics & Overall Health

Thinning hair may be caused by a genetic predisposition or a family history of thinning hair. Many times, this thinning is first noticed along the hairline. Health problems such as hyper- and hypothyroidism, medications and treatments such as chemotherapy, and hormone-replacement medications (including birth-control pills), are thinning-hair culprits

Overprocessing of Chemical Treatments

Chemical damage from overprocessing can also lead to thinning edges and eventually complete hair loss. The hairlines in the front and back of the head are the most delicate areas. These areas tend to process quickly, so great care should be exercised. Always follow manufacturer's instructions for chemical use to the letter. Of course, it's always best to have salon professionals handle chemical services whenever possible.

Finally, carefully monitor the use of chemicals in your hair care routine. Avoid double-processing the hair with bleach, permanent colors, perms or relaxers whenever possible.

Intervention & Preventing Relapse
Styling Choices

Unfortunately, the damage from constant thinning can be irreversible. If proper measures

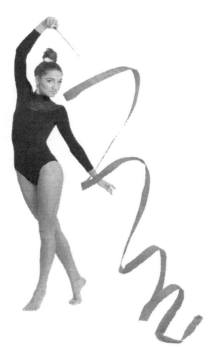

Figure 158- Dancers, gymnasts, and other female athletes often wear sleek styles that put a lot of pressure on the hairline.

that may also initially trigger thinning along the hairline.

Thinning hair can sometimes be attributed to poor eating habits and a lack of key minerals such as iron in the blood. Diet and medical issues should always be ruled out and addressed promptly.

Physical Abuse

High-heat styling routines almost always lead to thinning hair around the edges and elsewhere. Hair around the frontal hairline is often finer than the hair farther back from the face. The heat tolerance for this hair is also much lower.

If you are finding that the hair along your back hairline or nape area is thinning, check your winter gear! Wool and cotton hats, scarves and coats may be rubbing away your hair!

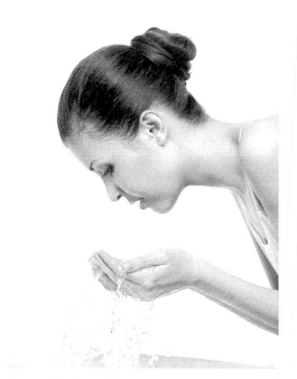

Figure 159- Facial cleansers can be especially hard on the finer hair that frames your face.

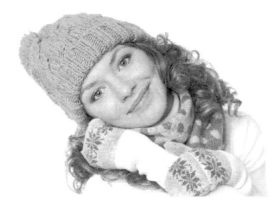

Figure 160- Turtlenecks, scarves, coats, and other winter gear can rub and break hair on the back hairline.

aren't taken to correct the issue immediately, permanent damage and hair loss from traction alopecia may result. The hairline is naturally finer than the bulk of the scalp hair, so it is best to wear styles that do not put tension on these finer, thinner areas. Flowing styles, loosely gathered styles, and other free-movement styles are great for this.

Loosen ponytails and other gathered styles to ensure that there is no tension or pulling at any point. To test your tension: Gather your hair into your intended ponytail but, just before securing it with the holder, bend your head down until your chin touches your chest. Check for tension and pulling. Then, slowly roll your head from side to side. If you feel even the slightest tug, loosen your grip. As a rule of thumb, avoid circling your ponytail with the holder more than two or three times when you secure it.

If you have pronounced thinning around the frontal hairline, try wearing face-framing bangs to take tension off the sparse areas and give the hair there a chance to make a comeback!

Scalp Massages

Consider massaging your scalp twice a day in your thinner areas. For an added benefit, use essential oils such as peppermint and rosemary to stimulate your scalp. The oils will improve circulation to your scalp in the massaged areas, and encourage a healthy scalp environment. Adding these stimulating oils to your shampoo or conditioner may help you as well.

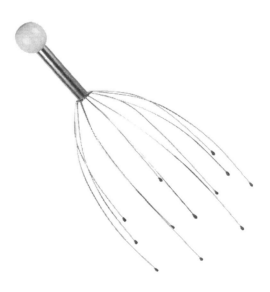

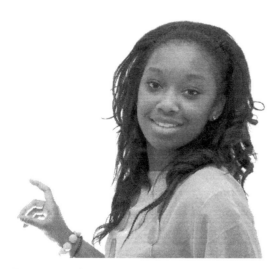

Figure 161- Chemical overprocessing almost always leads to thinning hair edges.

Figure 162- Scalp massage can help improve circulation to sparse areas. The scalp massager pictured here is easy on the scalp.

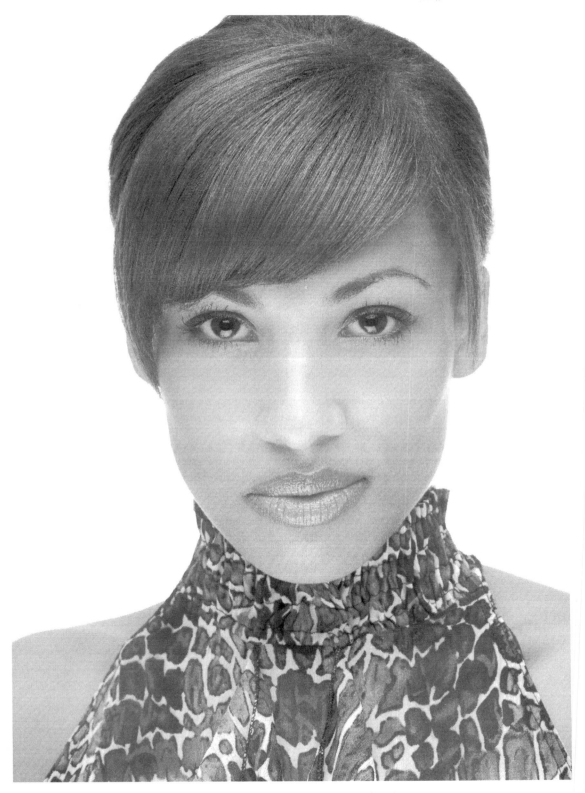

Figure 163- Bangs can help relieve tension on a stressed-out hairline.

Thin Ends

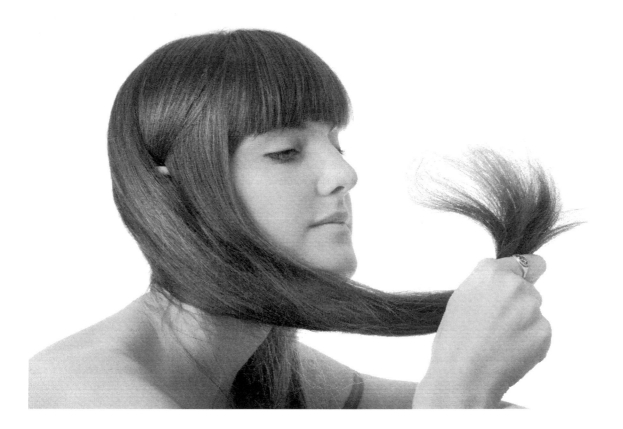

Is your hair full and thick at the roots (and along much of the length) but eerily whisper-thin at the very ends? Thinning ends are a natural feature of long, healthy hair that is rarely trimmed to neaten the ends. But when such thinning impacts individuals with much shorter hair lengths (i.e., just below the shoulder and shorter) and those who do maintain their hair with trimming, there is often a problem. Before you start trimming your ends, you should pinpoint the exact cause of your thinning. If your thinning has been ushered in by damage, the tips in this section will help you regain your hair's thickness at the ends.

Signs & Symptoms

Ends that taper in thickness and do not seem to accumulate length over time are a sign of unresolved hair damage and hair stress. This hair stress can be natural wear and tear or simply brought on by poor hair care practices. Signs and symptoms include:

- Excessive hair thinning near the ends.
- Limp or wispy, flyaway hair.
- Chronic hair breakage.

Causes & Triggers

The major causes of hair thinning at the very ends of our hair are:

- Natural weathering.
- Mechanical breakage.
- Heat use.
- Chemical overprocessing.

Natural Weathering

Hair, like most things in life, gets old and starts to show its age over time. The primary trigger for hair thinning at the ends, especially in longer hair, is natural weathering. The hair that is closest to the scalp is younger, healthier hair—but as we move down long strands, hair naturally becomes older, more ragged, and worn. This hair has seen more shampooings, more conditionings, more brushings, and more handling than the hair that has recently come in at the roots—and it just naturally tapers in response.

A second reason for natural thinning in longer hair is that individual strands in a head of longer hair are also more likely to have reached the end of their natural growing phases. Since each hair is on its own growth clock, it is not uncommon for hairs to naturally vary in length as new hairs start their growth cycle and older strands fall. This natural cycling of hair gives the appearance of thinning or tapering ends.

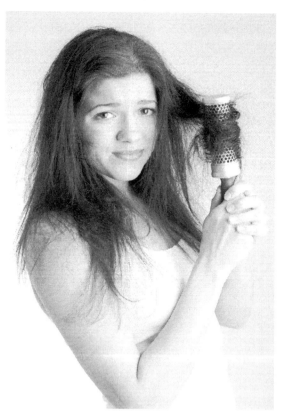

Figure 164- Mechanical breakage from combing and brushing is a common cause of thin ends.

For those with shorter hair, natural weathering also competes with a ton of other hair stressors. If the ends of the hair are not adequately protected from styling and environmental stressors, they will begin to thin out prematurely over time.

Mechanical Breakage

Many of the hair care tools we use every day to style our hair can lead to mechanical breakage and thinning problems. Combs, clips, hairpins, hairbands, and other tools with rough edges, serrated teeth, metal clasps and crimps, or springs-even rubber bands wrapped tightly around the ends of braids-can abrade the hair and lead to wispy ends.

Heat Use

Regular heat use is one of the main causes of hair thinning near the ends of the shaft. Heat throws off the moisture balance within the hair strand. Because the ends of the hair tend to be more porous and have comparatively less intact protein infrastructure to retain moisture, severe breakage and splitting occurs at the ends of the hair shaft with heat use.

Overprocessing from Overlapping

When chemical treatments are reapplied to the hair, there is an increased chance for overlapping onto previously treated hair. Over time, this weakens the hair fiber and speeds the natural weathering of the hair strand, resulting in thinner strands.

Intervention & Preventing Relapse

The simple solution for thinning ends is to just trim the hair so that the ends appear fuller. You may opt to clip them all in one sitting or gradually over the course of time to preserve your current length. This works for hair that is already healthy and only tapering due to wear and tear. For those who are battling damage, trimming the damage is only the first step. The next step should be identifying the primary cause of the damage and eliminating it from the regimen once and for all.

Low-Heat Regimen

Protective styling measures are important for keeping thinning ends to a minimum. Try going on a low-heat regimen, using direct heat on the hair no more than twice per month. If that sounds like an unbelievable stretch, or if you are a daily heat abuser, try weaning yourself down to

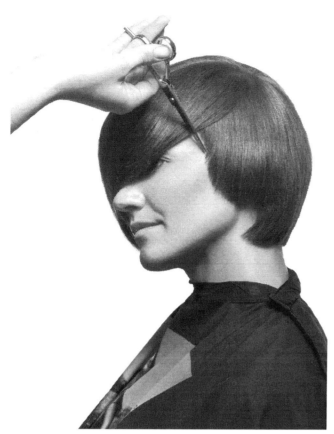

Figure 165- The easiest fix for thinning ends is to simply cut the thinning hair.

Backpack, shoulderbag, and purse straps can also tangle and damage the ends of the hair. Cotton and wool clothes, jackets, and scarves are great moisture absorbers. If your hair is constantly catching and rubbing against these fabrics each day, then thin ends can quickly become a problem. The trauma of rubbing roughs up the cuticle and begins to chip, fracture, and break down its protective covering.

Thin ends can also become a problem when the hair is constantly exposed to the elements. Bitter cold and scorching hot temperatures, wind, and surf can also degrade the cuticle and damage the precious ends.

heat once or twice per week at first. The finer or curlier your hair is, the lower its heat tolerance. With this regimen, you really need to focus on the last two to three inches of hair, keeping them moisturized and protected at all times.

Prevent Overprocessing

The best ways to guard against thinning from chemical overprocessing is to treat only hair that is in tip-top condition and only for the manufacturer's suggested processing time for your hair type. Ensure that you have adequate new growth or "roots" to allow for a safe touch-up application. Spacing treatments eight weeks apart or more usually ensures there is enough new hair growth to prevent overlapping.

If you are chemically relaxing the hair, coat the hair ends with oil or a petroleum-based product before application. When you rinse the relaxer, the ends of the hair will be shielded from further chemical exposure.

Moisturize & Protect

Be diligent about keeping your ends moisturized and protected. Deep condition your ends on a schedule that works for you—once a week generally works for most hair types.

Apply moisturizers to the ends (last two to three inches of hair) first, and then apply them to the rest of your hair. The ends are the oldest parts of the hair; with age, your hair is less able to retain moisture on its own. If your hair is thick or coarse, it may benefit from application of a light oil product after your moisturizer to give it some staying power. If your hair is fine or straight, you can skip this additional sealing step to prevent your hair from going too limp. The key is to never allow your hair to dry out. Once the hair's moisture and elasticity decrease dramatically, breakage, cracking, and tearing of the hair cuticle can occur. Finally, keep your hair in styles that protect your ends from the elements.

Unit IV:
Outpatient Therapy

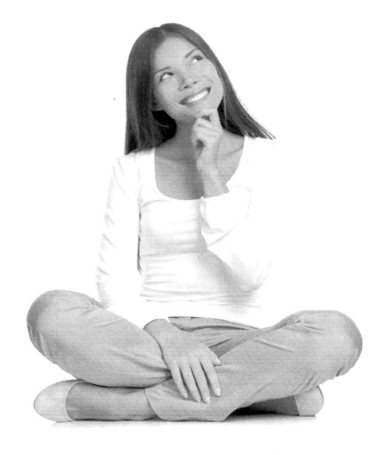

Chapter 7:

Special Hair Conditioning & Restoration Treatments

This section is dedicated to common home remedies and special hair conditioning and hair restoration treatments. Over the years, the green and back-to-nature movements have led to an increase in the number of people who've decided to take product creation into their own hands. There are several centuries-old remedies (and modern spin-offs of these remedies) widely accessible today on the web with one simple click of the mouse. We've compiled some of our favorite natural remedies here, along with some tweaks and personal touches that have proven useful.

Although the remedies and recipes in this section are made of natural ingredients and products from around the house, you should check to be sure that you are not allergic to any of the ingredients by performing a skin test prior to using them. Don't feel you're held hostage by the ingredients list—it's flexible and just there to guide you. Feel free to make any personal changes you need to make the recipe work for your situation. The most important thing to do is experiment. Vary the ingredients to customize the treatment recipes to your hair.

Hair & Scalp Treatment Building Blocks

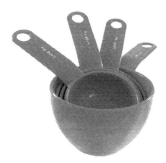

Figure 166- Break out the measuring cups for your homemade treatment lab.

If you are the adventurous type, building your own conditioning treatment may be the next best thing to those hard-to-gauge, off-the-shelf products for improving your hair. Once you know the benefits of different types of product ingredients, you can build your own perfect treatment from scratch—or take an existing product that you love as a base, and custom fit it for your needs. Go ahead: Open your cupboards and refrigerators! There's a wealth of healthy hair care treatment options inside!

Keep in mind that many homemade hair treatments have expiration dates because of the perishable items often used to create them. If you are creating a mixture that contains water or milk, for instance, the product will need to be refrigerated and used up completely (usually in three to four days). Without preserving your mixture, harmful bacteria, fungi, mold, and yeast may grow in your homemade product. Adding a natural preservative such as salt or an essential oil to your hair treatment may prolong its life.

Basic Ingredients You'll Want On Hand

If you are not sure which ingredients to include in your mixture, it's helpful to first determine your product's goal. *Do you want a cleanser? Or something to detangle your hair and provide moisture?* The list below categorizes common kitchen products by their hair benefits. Product customization becomes quite easy when you understand the characteristics and purpose of each common ingredient.

For Cleansing
- Baking soda (pH 8.3 to 9.1)
- Bentonite clay (pH 8.3 to 9.1)
- Lemon juice (pH 2.0 to 3.0)
- Apple cider vinegar (pH 2.5 to3.5)

For Moisture & Hydration

- Aloe vera (pH 4.0)
- Water (pH 7.0)
- Glycerin (pH 6.0-8.0)
- Honey (pH 3.2 -4.5)

For Protein & Structure
- Eggs
- Gelatin

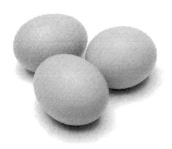

- Banana
- Avocado

For Smoothing, Sealing & Treatment Consistency

- Shea butter
- Vegetable oil
- Olive oil
- Coconut oil
- Castor oil
- Mayonnaise

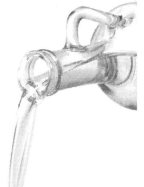

For Shine Enhancement

- Lemon juice (pH 2.0 to 3.0)
- Apple cider vinegar (pH 2.5-3.5)

Preservation, Scent & Sensory Effects

Several drops of the following essential oils can be added to homemade treatments and even to off-the-shelf shampoos, conditioners, and moisturizers to help preserve them (in the case of homemade products), improve their scent, boost their potency, and achieve particular scalp and hair benefits.

WARNING: Pregnant women, those who are nursing, and those with sensitive skin conditions should check with a medical practitioner prior to using essential oils on their hair or skin.

Essential Oils

- Cedarwood: Astringent/cleanser and dandruff-fighter.
- Jasmine: Scalp stimulant. Controls sebum production.
- Lavender: Soothes dry, itchy scalps.

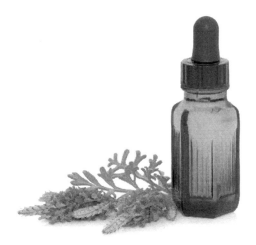

- Peppermint: Scalp stimulant. Great for soothing itchy, inflamed scalps.
- Rosemary: Scalp stimulant.
- Tea Tree: Scalp stimulant and dandruff-fighter. Controls sebum production. Thyme: Scalp stimulant.
- Ylang-ylang: Scalp stimulant. Controls sebum production.

Carrier Oils

- Almond
- Grapeseed
- Jojoba
- Olive
- Sesame
- Shea butter (melted)
- Soybean
- Sweet almond

For Preservation

The chemical preservatives in many off-the-shelf products allow them to keep for months or years in the store. Unfortunately, the same doesn't hold true for homemade concoctions, which like food, tend to go rancid rather quickly. If your product contains water or another liquid ingredient, it should be refrigerated promptly. While they cannot guarantee you months of use, the following ingredients may extend the shelf life of your homemade treatments for several days to a week if your concoction is stored properly:

- Rosemary essential oil
- Jojoba oil
- Vitamin E oil
- Salt
- Lemon juice
- Vinegar
- Sugar

For best results, always make your mixtures in small, preferably one-use batches rather than in huge tubs or containers. Smaller batches will eliminate the need for preservation because your mixtures will be used quickly. Avoid exposing your mixture to direct sunlight, open air, heat, and germs from your hands as these will quickly make your mixture go rancid.

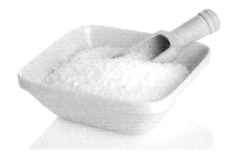

Figure 167- Salt is a common preservative.

Pre-shampoo Treatments
Island Breeze Pre-shampoo Treatment

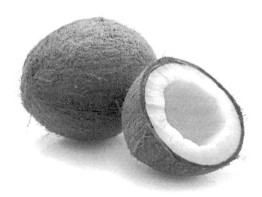

Figure 168- The properties of coconut can naturally improve the hair's elasticity.

Looking for a natural way to boost your hair's moisture levels? Try this simple pre-shampoo mix before your next wash. It smells great and will help improve moisture levels in your hair.

This Treatment

- Increases moisture levels within the hair.
- Softens hair.
- Improves elasticity.

You'll Need

- 1/2 cup instant conditioner (Suave and VO5 work great, or use your favorite)
- 1/2 can coconut milk (optional)
- 2 tablespoons oil (jojoba or sweet almond oil recommended)
- 2 tablespoons honey

Directions

Combine conditioner, coconut milk, oil, and honey and stir in a microwavable bowl. Warm the mixture in the microwave at 10-second intervals until the treatment reaches the desired warmth. Thoroughly rinse hair in warm water. Apply concoction to your damp hair in sections. Cover the hair with a plastic cap for 20 to 30 minutes. Rinse, and shampoo the hair as normal.

Caramel Hair Softener

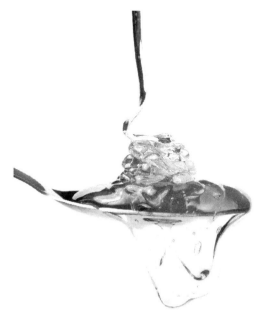

Figure 169- Caramel is an excellent softener for coarser hair types.

Caramel is certainly delicious to eat, but yes—you've guessed it—it works exceptionally well on your hair too! Caramel treatments are softness-boosting treatments. For curly girls, they can also lengthen curls and improve definition. These ultra-hydrating treatments are great for chemically-treated hair, and results can last anywhere from two to four weeks. Reserve this treatment for a day when you've got a little "me" time.

This Treatment

- Softens and hydrates hair.
- Makes frizzy hair smooth.
- Strengthens hair.

You'll Need

- 1/2 cup molasses or maple syrup
- 1/4 cup olive oil
- 4 tablespoons honey
- 2 bananas
- 1/2 cup water
- 4 tablespoons lemon juice
- 2 tablespoons all-purpose flour

Directions

Mix all ingredients until smooth. Ideally, you'll want to blend the banana in a mixer or blender to eliminate lumps. Gently warm the mixture on the stovetop. Warming the mixture will cause it to thicken slightly, but feel free to add or decrease the amount of flour (or water) to get the thickness you desire. Watch the mixture carefully. You want the treatment to be warm enough to comfortably apply to the hair but not hot enough to scald. Carefully spoon out some of the mixture and test by placing a small amount of the treatment on the back of your hand. The mixture will have a caramel color.

Separate your hair into four sections, and apply the caramel mixture to your hair. Cover your hair with a plastic conditioning cap and allow the mixture to sit for 45 minutes to 1 ½ hours. Treatment time depends upon the hair's level of dryness. Thoroughly rinse the mixture from your hair. Shampoo with a gentle, sulfate-free shampoo and proceed to deep condition for another 10 minutes or as needed.

Gentle Cleansing & Clarifying Treatments

Apple Cider Vinegar Rinse

Residues and buildup from shampoos, conditioners, and even your tap water can take the gorgeous glow from your hair. The apple cider vinegar rinse is an age-old treatment that is perfect for those who wish to reduce their hair's

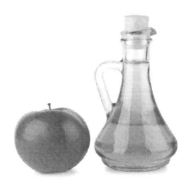

Figure 170- Apple cider vinegar naturally boosts hair's sheen and shine.

porosity and quickly boost its sheen and shine. Others may use apple cider vinegar to cleanse their hair in place of shampoo. Either way, apple cider vinegar rinsing can get you fast results!

This Treatment

- Adds shine.
- Gives hair a clean feel.
- Reduces hair porosity.
- Balances the pH of hair and scalp.

You'll Need

- 1/2 cup apple cider vinegar
- 1 to 2 cups water

Directions

Combine apple cider vinegar with water in a large cup to dilute it.

To use as a cleanser: Rinse hair thoroughly with warm water to start the cleansing process. Carefully pour the mixture over your hair while gently massaging the scalp and hair. Follow with a light moisturizing conditioner if desired to restore the hair's elasticity.

To use as a finisher, sealer, and shine booster: Use cool/cold water, and pour the mixture over the hair after rinsing out your conditioner. Lightly rinse the hair in cool water to remove any lingering vinegar odor. Dry and style your hair as normal.

Baking Soda Power Cleanse

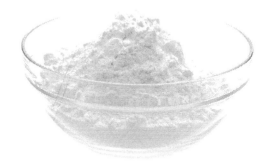

Figure 171- Baking soda can be a harsh yet effective cleanser.

Baking soda has been used as a household cleanser for ages. This non-lathering cleanser is also making waves as a hair cleanser, particularly for those who have forgone traditional shampoos in favor of all-natural products.

This Treatment

* Removes product buildup from hair.

You'll Need

* 2 cups warm water or 1/3 cup shampoo (your favorite)
* 1 to 2 tablespoons baking soda

Directions

Combine water (or shampoo) with baking soda. Stir the mixture well, ensuring that most of the baking soda dissolves in the water.

Rinse your hair thoroughly with warm water for several minutes. Pour the baking soda mixture over your head and hair. Gently massage the mixture into your scalp, and allow it to sit for a few minutes. (Baking soda rinses the hair clean but does not produce bubbles or lather. It can also make the hair feel a bit gritty, especially if it is not well dissolved in the water. If this bothers you, adding a tablespoon or two of baking soda to your shampoo instead of to plain water may help.) Rinse your hair, ensuring that all gritty particles are removed.

NOTE: The grittiness and high pH of baking soda may cause issues with cuticle abrasion. While many people regularly use baking soda on the hair without problems, be sure that your baking soda is properly diluted and dissolved and that your hair's pH is brought down to the normal 4 to 5.5 range with a conditioner or acidic rinse after use.

Bentonite Clay Mask

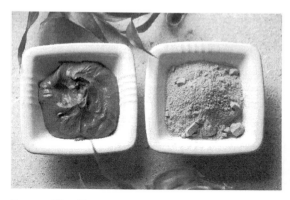

Figure 172- Clay is an age-old remedy for naturally cleansing the hair.

Bentonite clay is an excellent skin cleanser and has been used to alleviate and clear up skin issues ranging from simple acne to scalp problems such as eczema and psoriasis. This clay improves skin circulation and rejuvenates tired skin, which is a bonus for overworked scalps!

This Treatment

- Removes product buildup from hair.
- Detangles hair.
- Softens hair.
- Makes natural curls and waves pop or spring to life.

You'll Need

- 1 cup Bentonite clay powder
- 2 cups warm water or coconut milk
- 1/2 cup olive oil
- 1 to 2 tablespoons honey (optional)

Directions

After putting Bentonite clay powder in a bowl, slowly add warm water and olive oil until the mixture is the consistency of cake batter. For a bare-basics mixture, use clay and water only. If more conditioning is desired, fold in a little honey.

Thoroughly rinse your hair with warm water to remove debris. Apply the clay mixture to the hair in sections. Once fully applied, allow the clay to sit on the hair for approximately fifteen minutes. Do not allow the clay to dry on the hair. Rinse thoroughly in cool water.

Lemon-Squeeze Cleanser

Unleash the power of lemon in this wonderfully refreshing lemon clarifying rinse.

This Treatment

- Gently removes product buildup from hair.

You'll Need

- 1/2 cup fresh lemon juice
- 2 tablespoons honey
- 2 cups warm water

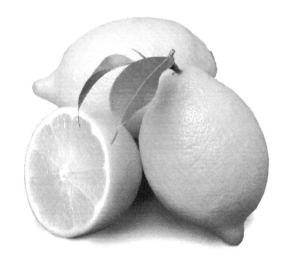

Figure 173- A touch of lemon is all that is needed in this refreshing cleansing recipe.

- 1 to 2 tablespoons baking soda (optional)

Directions

Combine all ingredients and mix well to ensure baking soda is dissolved (if used).

Thoroughly rinse hair in warm water to loosen product buildup. Pour the lemon rinse over the hair. (Include baking soda in the mixture for a deeper, more powerful cleansing.)

Dry Cocoa Shampoo

Just out of the gym or simply need to refresh your 'do before your regular shampoo? Try this homemade dry shampoo. Old-fashioned cocoa and cornstarch are the stars of this recipe. Give it a go!

This Treatment

- Gently absorbs sweat, oil and odors from hair between regular cleansings.

You'll Need

- 1/4 cup cocoa powder (or cornstarch or unscented baby powder)

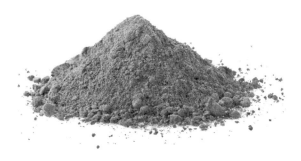

Figure 174- Cocoa powder's fine grains are great for absorbing oil and "dry cleaning" the hair.

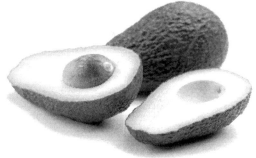

Figure 175- Avocado is a natural way to condition stressed-out strands.

Directions

Pour the powder into the palm of one hand and use the fingers of your other hand to apply the treatment. Using just the pads of your fingers, apply the powder to the scalp and roots of your hair only. Part the hair to expose the areas most plagued by oil. Massage and work the powder into the scalp until the excess oil has been absorbed. Gently brush the powder out of the hair.

HINT: Feel free to use the powdered product that works best for you! Cocoa blends better on darker hair, but those with lighter colored hair can use it too! Cornstarch and baby powder work best for those with light-colored hair, but a good brushing at the end will make those powders work well on darker hair too.

Conditioning Treatments & Packs

Avocado Hair Mask

In this recipe, avocados combine with eggs to make a magnificent hair and scalp conditioning treatment. Avocado-based treatments are great for hydrating parched hair in the hot summer months.

This Treatment

- Conditions the hair.
- Improves elasticity.
- Hydrates dry, flaky scalps.

You'll Need

- 1 or 2 ripe avocados
- 1 egg yolk
- 1 tablespoon olive oil or almond oil
- 1 tablespoon honey

Directions

Cut the avocado in half, and remove the seed. Use a spoon to scoop out the avocado pulp and mash it into a creamy paste. Add the egg yolk, honey, and oil, and mix well.

Rinse hair in warm water to lift and remove debris. Section the hair and apply the mask to the lower 4 inches and the ends of the hair first. Then apply the mask higher up the shaft and over the scalp. Cover with a plastic cap for 15 to 20 minutes. Rinse in cool water, and follow with a conditioner if desired.

Banana Power Conditioning Mask

Have a few bananas that are starting to go brown? Before you throw them away, try this great natural recipe! This treatment can also be used as a pre-shampoo treatment.

This Treatment

- Conditions the hair.

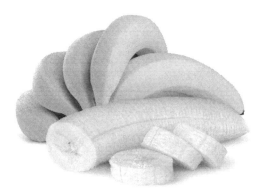

Figure 176- Bananas pack a light protein punch that will strengthen weak tresses.

- Improves elasticity.
- Hydrates dry, flaky scalps.
- Moisturizes dry or coarse hair.

You'll Need

- 1 or 2 ripe bananas
- 1 to 2 tablespoons honey
- 1 tablespoon olive or almond oil
- 2 to 3 drops lavender oil

Directions

Mix together banana and honey and blend into a smooth puree. (The puree should be liquid and contain no lumps of banana. Any lumps will be extremely difficult to rinse clean.) Add olive or almond oil and the lavender. Saturate the hair with warm water and apply your Banana Power Conditioning Mask. For extra penetration, place a plastic shower cap over your head and wrap your head with a warmed towel. Allow the mask to penetrate the hair for at least 15 minutes. Rinse thoroughly.

Cucumber Paradise Conditioning Mask

Cucumbers are packed with water (almost 96 percent) and are an excellent source of vitamins A and C, potassium, sulfur, and some B complex vitamins. Cucumber has been used in the treatment of eczema, psoriasis, and acne because of its soothing properties.

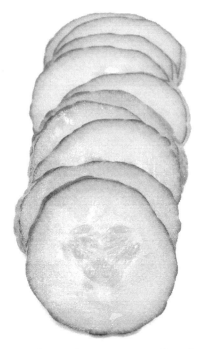

Figure 177- Cucumber is an excellent hair hydrator.

This Treatment

- Conditions the hair.
- Improves elasticity.
- Moisturizes dry, damaged hair.

You'll Need

- 2 peeled cucumbers
- 3 tablespoons honey
- ½ cup aloe vera gel
- 1 tablespoon olive oil or almond oil

Directions

Combine peeled cucumbers, honey, aloe vera gel, and oil, and blend into a smooth puree. Apply to the hair for 15 minutes. Rinse in warm water and proceed to the conditioning stage. This treatment can also be done as a pre-shampoo treatment.

Coconut Crème Conditioner

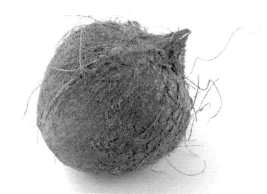

Figure 178- The coconut oil in this creamy conditioner improves elasticity.

Coconut is an amazing conditioner for all hair types. It reduces stress and strain on hair when used during cleansing and drying, and also helps to fortify and bind moisture to the hair.

This Treatment

- Conditions the hair.
- Improves elasticity.
- Moisturizes dry, damaged hair.

You'll Need

- 4 tablespoons conditioner (your favorite or an inexpensive brand such as VO5 or Suave)
- 2 tablespoons coconut oil
- 2 tablespoons olive oil or almond oil
- 2 to 3 drops lavender oil

Directions

Combine all ingredients in a bowl, and gently warm in the microwave. Alternatively, if you bottle the mixture, place the bottle in the shower to warm while you bathe and wash your hair. Carefully squeeze excess water from your hair, and apply the conditioner mixture liberally, focusing on the ends of the hair. Allow the mixture to stay in the hair for 10 to 15 minutes. Rinse thoroughly in cool water.

Protein Treatments & Packs
Protein Smoothie

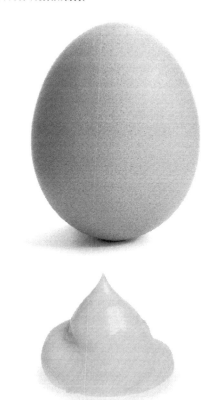

Figure 179- Eggs and mayonnaise combine in this recipe to strengthen and condition the hair.

You can make your own protein "smoothie" treatment by whipping up simple ingredients from your refrigerator! This particular treatment is a mild to moderately strong protein treatment, depending upon the ingredient ratios you use.

This Treatment

- Adds shine.
- Adds thickness and volume.
- Strengthens hair.
- Reduces frizz.

You'll Need

- 2 egg yolks
- 1/2 cup mayonnaise
- 2 to 3 tablespoons honey
- 3/4 cup conditioner (your choice)
- 1 tablespoon olive oil or other oil of your choice

Directions

Combine eggs, mayonnaise, honey, conditioner and oil in a bowl and blend until smooth. You may play around with the measurements for this smoothie to suit your needs. Just be sure to have some form of protein (i.e. eggs) and a conditioning agent (honey, olive oil, or conditioner). A simpler version of this recipe, for instance, uses only eggs and olive oil.

Apply the treatment to your hair for 20 to 30 minutes. At the end of the treatment, rinse with cool water. Be sure that you deep condition very well following the treatment because the protein may make your hair harder (stronger) and somewhat harder to detangle without conditioning support.

Banana Pudding Protein Mask

The Banana Mash Protein Mask is a spin-off of the Protein Smoothie, except that it

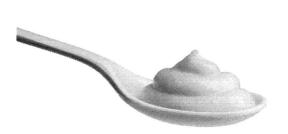

Figure 180- Try this banana protein mask to fortify the hair.

contains amino acid–rich sweet bananas. Bananas also contain a plethora of natural oils that are considered to be extremely beneficial to the health of hair and skin. The banana component of this treatment increases the elasticity of your hair and balances the strengthening properties of the egg. This mask treatment provides a moderate to high level of protein. You may play around with the measurements to suit your own tastes.

This Treatment

- Adds shine.
- Adds thickness and volume.
- Strengthens hair.

You'll Need

- 2 egg yolks
- 2 ripe bananas
- 2 to 3 tablespoons honey
- 1/2 cup conditioner (coconut-scented)
- 2 tablespoons olive oil (or oil of your choice)

Directions

Put all ingredients in a blender or food processor and mix until the bananas are well pureed. (The puree should be liquid and contain no lumps of banana. Any lumps will be extremely difficult to rinse clean.)

Apply the treatment to your hair for 20 to 30 minutes. Rinse with cool water. Your hair will feel very strong and thick and have great shine! If you are using this treatment solely for supplemental protein, be sure that you deep condition very well following the treatment. The protein may make your hair harder (stronger) and somewhat harder to detangle without conditioning support.

To thicken fine hair: This treatment works extremely well for those with fine, thin hair. If using this treatment to enhance thickness, you may opt to skip the deep conditioning, and simply do a 2 to 3 minute rinse with a light detangling conditioner. A heavier conditioner will weigh the hair down and return the hair to its original thinner appearance.

Other Treatments
Ocean Spray

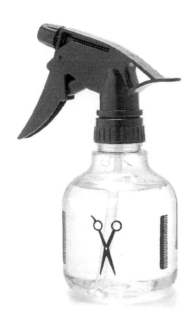

Figure 181- A mister bottle works great for water-based moisture products on the go.

If you love the amazing softness, texture, and body that comes from swimming out at sea—you'll love this quick and easy knock-off spray.

This Treatment

- Adds body, volume and texture.

You'll Need

- 1 tablespoon Epsom salts
- 1 to 2 tablespoons conditioner (your favorite)
- 1 cup warm water

Directions

Shake all ingredients together in a spritz bottle. Mist onto already damp or dry hair. Scrunch and work fingers through the hair to bring on texture and waves.

Add more water or conditioner to increase the moisture in this mixture—or to accommodate longer or thicker hair. For more defined texture, add a dollop of hair gel to your mixture. Ingredients will settle, so shake well before each use.

Honey-Lime Coconut Curl Releaser

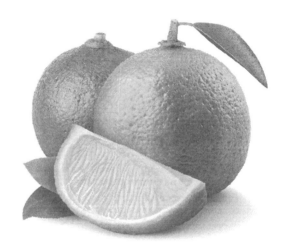

Figure 182- Try the Honey-Lime Curl Releaser to stretch and add sheen to your curly hair.

For those of you who wish to lengthen and define your curls, this temporary Honey-Lime Coconut Curl Releaser may help. The powerful properties of lime, honey, and coconut in combination temporarily loosen and define tightly curled hair naturally. Give this one a try!

This Treatment

- Lengthens and stretches curls.
- Adds shine and sheen.

You'll Need

1 15-ounce (400 ml) can coconut milk
1/4 cup lime or lemon juice
1 tablespoon olive oil
2 tablespoons honey

Directions

Refrigerate the coconut milk and allow it to naturally separate. It will create a thick, creamy foam at the top. Spoon off the cream and place in a bowl. Add lime (or lemon) juice, olive oil, and honey, and stir well to blend.

Separate your hair into four sections, and then apply the cream to your hair. If your hair is chemically straightened, you may concentrate the cream on your new growth. (Alternatively, you may use a spray bottle to apply this mixture to your hair.) Cover your hair with a plastic conditioning cap, and allow the mixture to sit for 30 to 45 minutes. Thoroughly rinse the mixture from your hair and deep condition for another 10 minutes or as needed. Repeat once or twice a week as desired, and watch your hair gradually lengthen out!

Chapter 8:

On the Shelf!

Many of the treatments in the *Special Hair Conditioning & Restoration Treatments* section can easily be made at home, but if you're like most people, walking around smelling like mayonnaise and olive oil isn't that appealing. Maybe you just don't have time to mix random grocery store items together, and you'd rather spend your time eating avocados than wearing them as hair mask. Understandable.

Here's a list of some top products that may help you through your rehab regimen. No pressure—they are just here for guidance! This list isn't exhaustive, and some really great products aren't listed because, well—this book would have become a dictionary! Do a little research and see what works for you! We are all different, and what works for you may not work for your mom, sister, or friend with the same hair type—even if the experts say it should. That's why there are so many products out on the market today—there is hardly a consensus on what works!

The products listed below span the price range from low end to high end. Some products are even organic—if that's your thing. All of these products can be picked up either in your local beauty supply store or from beauty outlets such as ULTA and Sephora, drugstores, Amazon.com (and other online retailers), most major large-chain retailers, and salons all over.

Shampoos

Chelating Shampoos

WHEN TO USE: In Rehab Step 1, after swimming, or monthly for basic anti–hard water maintenance. For extreme hard-water cases, use a gentle chelating shampoo every 1 to 2 weeks to control mineral buildup.

Alba Botanica Daily Shampoo
Artec Texturline Daily Clarifying Shampoo
Bumble and Bumble Sunday Shampoo
Curl Junkie Daily Fix Cleanser
Elucence Moisture Acidifying Shampoo
Joico Resolve Chelating Shampoo
Kenra Clarifying Shampoo

KeraCare DeMineralizing Treatment
Nexxus Aloe Rid Gentle Clarifying Shampoo
Nexxus Phyto Organics Kelate Purifying Shampoo
Ouidad Water Works Shampoo
Paul Mitchell Shampoo Three
Pureology Purify Shampoo
Redken Hair Cleansing Cream Shampoo

Clarifying Shampoos

WHEN TO USE: In Rehab Step 1 (optional-instead of chelating shampoo), monthly for basic product-buildup removal, or as needed for fine or oily hair.

Alba Botanica Daily Shampoo
Alterna Clarifying Shampoo
Aubrey Organics Green Tea Clarifying Shampoo
Avalon Organics Clarifying Lemon Shampoo
Bumble and Bumble Sunday Shampoo
Carol's Daughter Rosemary Mint Purifying
    Shampoo
CURLS Pure Curls Clarifying Shampoo
Elucence Volume Clarifying Shampoo
Hair Rules Aloe Grapefruit Purifying Shampoo
Jessicurl Gentle Lather Shampoo
Karen's Body Beautiful Cool Clarifying Shampoo
Kenra Clarifying Shampoo
Kiss My Face Aromatherapeutic Shampoo
Ouidad Clear & Gentle Essential Daily
    Shampoo
Redken Nature's Rescue Refreshing Detox
    Shampoo

NOTE: For gentle clarifying, most sulfate shampoos fall under this category.

Sulfate-Free Gentle Cleansing Shampoos
WHEN TO USE: In Rehab Step I after chelating shampoo, and from there onward. These gentle formulas work well for most types of hair, but if your hair is fine or oily, you may need products that volumize your hair as they gently clean.

Abba Pure Gentle Shampoo
Abba Pure Moisture Shampoo
Abba Pure Basic Shampoo
Abba Pure Color Protect Shampoo
Abba Pure Curl Shampoo
AG Hair Cosmetics Recoil Curl Activating
    Shampoo
Alba Botanica Cocoa Butter Shampoo
Alba Botanica Coconut Milk Shampoo
Alba Botanica Gardenia Shampoo
Alba Botanica Honeydew Shampoo
Alba Botanica Plumeria Shampoo
Alba Botanica Daily Shampoo

Alterna Bamboo Luminous Shine Shampoo
Alterna Bamboo Smooth Anti-Frizz Shampoo
Anita Grant Babassu Amla Shampoo Bar
Anita Grant Babassu Lavender Rose Shampoo
    Bar
Anita Grant Peppermint Babassu Shampoo
    Bar
Anita Grant Organic Kelp + Ylangylang
    Babassu Shampoo Bar
Aubrey Organics BGA Protein +
    Strengthening Shampoo
Aubrey Organics GPB Glycogen Protein
    Balancing Shampoo
Aubrey Organics Honeysuckle Rose
    Moisturizing Shampoo
Aubrey Organics Island Naturals Replenishing
    Shampoo
Aubrey Organics J.A.Y. Desert Herb
    Revitalizing Shampoo
Aubrey Organics Rosa Mosqueta Nourishing
    Shampoo
Aubrey Organics White Camellia Ultra
    Smoothing Shampoo
Avalon Organics Awapuhi Mango
    Moisturizing Shampoo
Avalon Organics Extra Moisturizing Olive
    and Grapeseed Shampoo
Avalon Organics Nourishing Lavender Shampoo
Avalon Organics Shine Ylang Ylang Shampoo
Avalon Organics Smoothing Grapefruit &
    Geranium Shampoo
Avalon Organics Strengthening Peppermint
    Shampoo
Avalon Organics Tea Tree Mint Treatment
    Shampoo
Avalon Organics Tea Tree Scalp Treatment
    Shampoo
Avalon Organics Tear-Free Baby Shampoo
Avalon Organics Volumizing Rosemary
    Shampoo
Aveda Scalp Benefits Balancing Shampoo
Aveda Damage Remedy Restructuring
    Shampoo

Aveda Dry Remedy Moisturizing Shampoo

Aveda Men's Pureformance Shampoo

Back to Basics Blue Lavender Color Protect Shampoo

Bed Head Foxy Curls Frizz-Fighting Sulfate-Free Shampoo

Bed Head Superstar Sulfate-Free Shampoo for Thick Massive Hair

Bee Mine Peppermint & Tea Tree Nourishing Shampoo

Blended Beauty Soy Cream Shampoo

Bumble and Bumble Straight Shampoo

Burt's Bees Baby Bee Shampoo & Wash

Burt's Bees Color Keeper Green Tea & Fennel Seed Shampoo

Burt's Bees More Moisture Raspberry & Brazil Nut Shampoo

Burt's Bees Rosemary Mint Shampoo Bar

Burt's Bees Super Shiny Grapefruit & Sugar Beet Shampoo

Curl Junkie Curl Assurance Gentle Cleansing Shampoo

CURLS Curlicious Curls Cleansing Cream Organic Shampoo

CUSH Hydration Supreme Conditioning Shampoo

DermOrganic Conditioning Shampoo

Design Essentials Natural Curl Cleanser Shampoo

DevaCurl No-Poo Cleanser

DevaCurl Low-Poo Cleanser

Elasta QP Creme Conditioning Shampoo

Elucence Moisture Benefits Shampoo

Giovanni Smooth as Silk Shampoo

Giovanni Tea Tree Triple Treat Shampoo

Giovanni 50:50 Balanced Shampoo

Giovanni Golden Wheat Shampoo

Giovanni Root 66 Max Volume

Giovanni Wellness Shampoo with Chinese Botanicals

Jane Carter Solution Hydrating Invigorating Shampoo

Jason Natural Aloe Vera Shampoo

Jason Natural Apricot Shampoo

Jason Natural Biotin Shampoo

Jason Natural Lavender Shampoo

Jason Natural Sea Kelp Moisturizing Shampoo

Jessicurl Hair Cleansing Cream Shampoo

Jonathan Product Weightless No Frizz Shampoo

Jonathan Product Hydrating Shampoo

Jonathan Product Green Routine Nourishing Shampoo

Karen's Body Beautiful Bodacious Beauty Bar

Karen's Body Beautiful Ultimate Conditioning Shampoo

Kenra Platinum Shampoo

KeraCare 1st Lather Shampoo

KeraCare Hydrating Detangling Shampoo

KeraCare Naturals Cleansing Cream

L'Oreal Everpure Smooth Shampoo

L'Oreal Everstrong Hydrating Shampoo

L'Oreal Everstrong Reconstructing Shampoo

MOP C-System Clean Shampoo

MOP C-System Hydrating Shampoo

Neutragena Triple Moisture Cream Lather Shampoo

Organix Awakening Mocho Expresso Shampoo

Organix Energizing Passion Fruit Guava Shampoo

Organix Enriching Cucumber Yogurt Shampoo

Organix Fortifying Lavender Soymilk Shampoo

Organix Healing Mandarin Olive Oil Shampoo

Organix Hydrating Tea Tree Mint Shampoo

Organix Instant Repair Cocoa Butter Shampoo

Organix Moisturizing Grapefruit Mango Butter

Organix Nourishing Coconut Milk Shampoo

Organix Nutritional Acai Berry Avocado Shampoo

Organix Rejuvenating Cherry Blossom Ginseng Shampoo

Organix Renewing Moroccan Argan Oil Shampoo

Organix Revitalizing Pomengranate Green
  Tea Shampoo
Organix Smoothing Shea Butter Shampoo
Organix Soft and Silky Vanilla Silk Shampoo
Oyin Grand Poo Bar
Pureology Essential Repair Shampoo
Pureology Hydrate Shampoo
Pureology Nanoworks Shampoo
Pureology Super Smooth Shampoo
Qhemet Biologics Egyptian Wheatgrass
  Cleansing Tea Shampoo
SheaMoisture Raw Shea Butter Moisture
  Retention Shampoo
Silk Elements ColorCare Sulfate-Free Shampoo
TIGI S-Factor Health Factor Sulfate-Free
  Daily Dose Shampoo
Trader Joe's Nourish Spa Shampoo
Trader Joe's Tea Tree Tingle Shampoo
WEN Cleansing Conditioner

**If the options above are too heavy or rich for
your oily or fine/ medium textured hair—try
these:**

Abba Volumizing Shampoo
Alba Botanica Daily Shampoo
Alba Botanica Hawaiian Shampoo- Body
  Builder Mango
Alterna Bamboo Abundant Volume Shampoo
Aubrey Organics Egyptian Henna Shine-
  Enhancing Shampoo
Avalon Organics Biotin B-Complex
  Thickening Shampoo
Avalon Organics Rosemary Volumizing
  Shampoo
Burt's Bees Very Volumizing Pomegranate &
  Soy Shampoo
Hair Rules Aloe Grapefruit Purifying
  Shampoo
Hair Rules Daily Cleansing Cream
Jason Vitamin E with A & C Shampoo
Jessicurl Gentle Lather Shampoo
Jonathan Product Infinite Volume Shampoo

Kinky-Curly Come Clean Moisturizing
  Shampoo
Kiss My Face Big Body Shampoo
L'Oreal Everpure Volumizing Shampoo
L'Oreal Everstrong Bodify Shampoo
Ouidad Clear & Gentle Essential Daily
  Shampoo
Pureology PureVolume Shampoo
Redken Nature's Rescue Refreshing Detox
  Shampoo

Conditioners
Moisture-Based Conditioners
Correcting hair dryness and breakage with
moisture conditioning is often necessary to
keep the hair in great shape. Used in the correct
frequency, the moisturizing conditioners listed
below will relieve dryness breakage due to low
moisture in the hair strands.

**Moisturizing Deep-Conditioning Products
WHEN TO USE:** In Rehab Step 2, and at least
once a week.

AtOne Botanicals Reconstructor w/ Moisture
  Recovery
Aubrey Organics Honeysuckle Rose Conditioner
Aubrey Organics Rosa Mosqueta Conditioner
Aubrey Organics White Camellia Conditioner
Aussie Moist Conditioner
Avalon Organics Awapuhi Mango
  Moisturizing Conditioner
Avalon Organics Lavender Nourishing
  Conditioner
Avalon Organics Ylangylang Glistening
  Conditioner
Aveda Dry Remedy Moisturizing Conditioner
Back to Basics Bamboo Straightening
  Conditioner
Back to Basics Rich Moisture Coconut Mango
Back to Basics Vanilla Plum Conditioner
Bee Mine Bee-U-Ti-Ful Deep Conditioner
Biolage Hydratherapie Conditioning Balm

Blended Beauty Herbal Reconditioner

Bumble and Bumble Seaweed Conditioner

Burt's Bees Super Shiny Grapefruit & Sugar Beet Conditioner

Curl Junkie Hibiscus & Banana Deep Fix Moisturizing Conditioner

Curl Junkie Curl Rehab Moisturizing Hair Treatment

Dove Advanced Care Sheer Moisture Conditioner

Dove Beautiful Care Conditioner

Dove Moisture Rich Color Conditioner

Dove Damage Therapy Daily Moisture Treatment

Elasta QP DPR-11 Deep Penetrating Remoisturizer

Elucence Moisture Balancing Conditioner

Frederic Fekkai Technician Color Care Conditioner

Frederic Fekkai Glossing Conditioner

Frederic Fekkai Luscious Curls Conditioner

Frederic Fekkai Shea Butter Moisturizing Conditioner

Giovanni Smooth as Silk Deeper Moisture Conditioner

Herbal Essences Hello Hydration Moisturizing Conditioner

Herbal Essences Color Me Happy Conditioner

Herbal Essences None of Your Frizzness Smoothing Conditioner

Herbal Essences Totally Twisted Curls and Waves Conditioner

Jane Carter Nutrient Replenishing Conditioner

JASON Plumeria & Sea Kelp Moisturizing Conditioner

Jessicurl Aloeba Daily Conditioner

Jessicurl Too Shea! Extra Moisturizing Conditioner

Jessicurl Weekly Deep Conditioning Treatment

Joico Moisture Recovery Conditioner

Joico Moisture Intensive Treatment Extra

Conditioning Conditioner

Kenra Moisturizing Conditioner

Kenra Nourishing Masque Deep Conditioning Treatment

Keracare Humecto Crème Conditioner

Keracare Moisturizing Conditioner for Color-Treated Hair

Kerastase Nutritive Masquintense Nourishing Treatment

Kinky Curly Knot Today Conditioner/ Detangler

L'Anza Healing ColorCare Color-Preserving Conditioner

Mizani Moisturefuse Moisturizing Conditioner

MOP C-System Moisture Complex Conditioner

MYHoneyChild Organic Shea Butter Hair Paste

MYHoneyChild SO DEEP Conditioner

MYHoneyChild Olive You Deep Conditioner

Neutragena Triple Moisture Daily Conditioner

Neutragena Triple Moisture Deep Recovery Mask

Nexxus Humectress Ultimate Moisturizing Conditioner

Nexxus Diametress Sublime Volume Luscious Bodifying Conditioner

Organix Nourishing Coconut Milk Conditioner

Organix Hydrating Tea Tree Mint Conditioner

Oyin Honey-Hemp Conditioner

Pantene Pro-V Color Preserve Smooth Conditioner

Redken Real Control Conditioner

Tigi Bed Head Moisture Maniac Conditioner

Trader Joe's Refresh Conditioner

If the options above are too heavy or rich for your oily or fine/medium textured hair—try these:

Aussie Aussome Volume Conditioner
Avalon Organics Biotin B-Complex
    Thickening Conditioner
Avalon Organics Rosemary Volumizing
    Conditioner
Aveda Color Conserve Conditioner
Back to Basics Apple Ginseng Volumizing
    Conditioner
Biolage Volumathérapie Full-Lift Volumizing
    Conditioner
Bumble and Bumble Seaweed Conditioner
Bumble and Bumble Thickening Conditioner
Herbal Essences BodyEnvy Volumizing
    Conditioner Jason Natural Biotin
    Conditioner
Jason Natural Sea Kelp Conditioner
Jason Natural Vitamin E with A & C
    Conditioner

Protein-Based Conditioners and Treatments

Protein conditioning is often necessary to balance
the moisturizing conditioning you are doing
and to keep the hair in great condition. Use the
products below a few times each month to give
your hair the strength and balance it needs.

Protein-Based Conditioners and Treatment Products

WHEN TO USE: In Rehab Step 2, every 2 to
6 weeks, or as needed.

Protein Products (Light/Flexible Strength)

Aubrey Organics Glycogen Protein Balancing
    (GPB) Conditioner
Aveda Damage Remedy Conditioner
Garnier Fructis Length & Strength Fortifying
    Cream Conditioner
Got2B Soft One Minute Emergency Repair
    Creme
Herbal Essences Long Term Relationship
    Conditioner
Joico Body Luxe Thickening Conditioner
Joico Moisture Recovery Treatment Balm

Joico K-Pak Reconstruct Conditioner
Mane and Tail Original Conditioner
Motions Moisture Silk Protein Conditioner
MYHoneyChild Banana Creme Conditioner
Neutrogena Triple Moisture Deep Recovery
    Mask
Organic Root Stimulator Replenishing Pak
Ovation Cell Therapy Crème Rinse
    Moisturizer
Paul Mitchell Super Strong Daily
    Conditioner
Phytospecific Intense Nutrition Mask
Redken Extreme Conditioner
Rusk Sensories Calm 60 Second Hair Revive
Trader Joes Nourish Spa Balance
    Moisturizing Conditioner
Vitale Pro Super Conditioner

Protein Products (Moderate Strength)

Aphogee Keratin 2 Minute Reconstructor
Elasta QP Breakage Control Serum
Elucence Extended Moisture Repair
    Treatment
Frederic Fekkai Protein Rx Reparative
    Conditioner
Giovanni Smooth As Silk Extreme Protein
    Treatment
LeKair Cholesterol Plus Strengthening
    Conditioning Cream
Motions Critical Protection and Repair (CPR)
    Treatment Conditioner
Nexxus Keraphix Restorative Strengthening
    Conditioner
Ovation Cell Therapy Conditioner Hair
    Treatment

Protein Products (Hard/Intense Strength)

Affirm 5 n I Reconstructor
Aphogee Two–Step Protein Treatment
Elasta QP Breakage Control Serum
Elucence Extended Moisture Repair
    Treatment
Joico K-Pac Deep Penetrating Reconstructor

Mizani Kerafuse Intensive Strengthening Treatment

Motions Critical Protection and Repair (CPR) Treatment Conditioner

Nexxus Emergencee Strengthening Polymeric Reconstructor

Nexxus Keraphix Restorative Strengthening Conditioner

Organic Root Stimulator Hair Mayonnaise Treatment for Damaged Hair

Shampoo & Conditioner Products for Color-Treated Hair

AG Hair Cosmetics Colour Savour Sulfate-free Shampoo & Conditioner

Biolage Colorcarethérapie Color Care Conditioner

CHI Ionic Color Protection System Sulfate Free Shampoo

Clairol Nice n' Easy ColorSeal Conditioner

Herbal Essences Color Me Happy Conditioner for Color-Treated Hair

Kenra Platinum Shampoo and Conditioner.

Pureology Hydrate Conditioner

RedKen Color Extend Conditioner

Leave-in Conditioners & Water-Based Moisturizers

Moisturizers are great to have in a hair care regimen, especially if your hair tends toward the dry side. If your hair is fine to medium, a leave-in conditioner spray or foam can provide all the moisture that is needed to keep the hair supple without weighing it down. If your hair is coarse or thick, you may benefit from both a leave-in conditioner and a separate creamy moisturizing product. The best water-based moisturizers do not contain heavy, hair shaft—coating oils such as mineral oil and petrolatum; rather, they contain a mixture of water, humectants, and natural oils or butters.

Leave-In & Water-Based Moisture Products (Moisture Focused)

WHEN TO USE: In Rehab Step 3, after hair is shampooed and conditioned, or every 1 to 3 days as needed for hydration. Those with very fine or oily hair may skip this layering step as needed.

Bumble and Bumble Leave-In Conditioner

Curl Junkie Hibiscus & Banana Honey Butta Leave-In

CURLS Curl Soufflé Organic Curl Cream

Giovanni Direct Leave-In Conditioner

Hair Rules Nourishment Leave In Conditioner

Herbal Essences None of Your Frizzness Leave-In

Herbal Essences Long Term Relationship Leave-In

It's a 10 Miracle Leave in Product

Jane Carter Solution Hair Nourishing Cream

Karen's Body Beautiful Hair Nectar

Kinky Curly Knot Today Leave-In Conditioner

Kenra Platinum Color Care Botanical Detangler

Kenra Daily Provision Leave-In Conditioner

L'ANZA Healing Moisture Leave-in Noni Fruit Detangler

L'ANZA Leave-In Conditioner

Neutragena Triple Moisture Silk Touch Leave-In Conditioner

Nexxus Humectress Luxe Moisturizing Leave-In Spray

Organic Root Stimulator (Carrot Oil) Moisturizer

Ouidad Botanical Boost Moisture Infusing & Refreshing Spray

Oyin's Frank Juice Nourishing Herbal Leave-In Conditioner

Oyin's Greg Juice Nourishing Herbal Leave-In Conditioner

Paul Mitchell The Detangler
Phytospecific Integral Hydrating Mist
Profectiv Damage Free Anti-Tangle Leave-In
Proline Lite Comb Thru Creme Moisturizer
SheaMoisture Organic Curl Enhancing
   Smoothie
Silk Elements MegaSilk Leave-In Hair
   Moisturizing Crème

Leave-Ins & Water-Based Moisture Products (Protein/Strengthening- Focused)
ApHogee Pro-Vitamin Leave-In Conditioner
ApHogee Green Tea Reconstructor
Cantu Shea Butter Break Cure Treatment
Cantu Shea Butter Grow Strong Treatment
Cantu Shea Butter Leave-In
Chi Keratin Mist
Elasta QP Mango Butter
Infusium 23 Leave-Ins
Profectiv Break Free Leave-In
Profectiv Break Thru Treatment
Profectiv Mega Growth Treatment
Profectiv Healthy Ends Treatment

Oils & Butters

Select one or more oils from the list. Fine to medium hair types may not need an oil to help the hair retain moisture. Lighter oil products may be used if needed or desired for the finest hair types.

Natural Oils
WHEN TO USE: In Rehab Step 4, after moisturizer to provide a seal for medium- to coarse-textured hair types that struggle with moisture retention.

Almond
Argan
Camellia (light)
Castor
Coconut (light)
Flaxseed

Jojoba (light)
Hemp
Moroccanoil Light (light)
Olive
Palm
Palm Kernel
Peanut
Safflower
Sesame
Soybean
Sunflower
Sweet Almond
Wheat Germ
Ximenia

Natural Butters
WHEN TO USE: In Rehab Step 4, and after moisturizer to provide a seal for medium to coarse/thick textured hair types that struggle with moisture retention.

Avocado
Cocoa
Coffee
Mango
Shea

Commercial Oil & Butter Products
WHEN TO USE: In Rehab Step 4, and after moisturizer to provide a seal for medium to coarse/thick textured hair types that struggle with moisture retention.

Carol's Daughter Healthy Hair Butter
CUSH Mango Pomade
Elasta QP Mango Butter
Dabur Vatika Oil
Dabur Amla Oil
Oyin Burnt Sugar Pomade
Oyin's Whipped Pudding

Ancillary Hair Products

Ancillary hair products are the products responsible for sculpting, smoothing, slicking, curl defining, and adding an extra bit of polish and control to our tresses. They can be optional, feel-good products—or absolute necessities for some people, depending on their style! These are just a few great products you can try and add to your hair care arsenal.

Dry Shampoos

WHEN TO USE: As needed. These powdered shampoos are great for perking up oily hair in between wash days and for hairstyles that can't be cleansed directly in water without ruining them.

Batiste Dry Shampoo
Got2b Rockin' It Dry Shampoo
John Frieda Luxurious Volume Refresher Dry
    Shampoo
Ojon Rub-Out Dry Cleanser
Pravana Fresh Volumizing Dry Shampoo
René Furterer Naturia Dry Shampoo
Tigi Rockaholic Dirty Secret Dry Shampoo
TRESemmé Fresh Start Waterless Foam
    Shampoo

Curl Creams and Gels

WHEN TO USE: As needed. These products help define and refresh curls and waves.

Aloe Vera Gel
Alterna Hemp Texturizing Glaze
Aveda Light Elements Defining Whip
Aubrey Organics Mandarin Magic Ginkgo
    Leaf and Ginseng Root Hair Jelly
Blended Beauty Curly Frizz Pudding
Blended Beauty Happy Nappy
Curl Junkie Aloe Fix Lite Hair Styling Gel
CURLS Curl Souffle Organic Curl Cream
CURLS Goddess Glaze Organic Gel
CURLS Whipped Cream

DevaCurl Set it Free
Ecostyler Gel
Fantasia IC Polisher with Sparklelites
Garnier Fructis Cream Gel
Jane Carter Solution Curl Defining Cream
Kinky Curly Curling Custard

Volumizing Mousses, Foams, and Root Lifters

WHEN TO USE: As needed. These products are great for building volume into limp or flat tresses.

Alterna Hemp Seed Thickening Compound
Aquage Uplifting Foam
Big Sexy Hair Root Pump PLUS – Humidity
    Resistant Volumizing Spray Mousse
Frizz-Eaze Take Charge Style-Managing
    Mousse
got2b Fat-Tastic Thickening Plumping
    Mousse
Kenra Volume Mousse
Paul Mitchell Lemon Sage Thickening Spray
Redken Body Full Instant Bodifier
Rusk Thick Body and Texture Amplifier
TIGI Catwalk Root Boost

Texturizing Pastes, Muds, Pomades & Waxes

WHEN TO USE: As needed. These finishing products mold, sculpt, and add texture, shine and definition to the hair—especially for shorter styles. Since they tend to be quite heavy, they can really weigh down fine to medium strands. (Finishing sprays are a better option for this group.) Pastes, muds, pomades, and waxes clump the strands together for a texturized, "piecey" or second-day hair look. Waxes are the heaviest texturizing products in the finishing group, while pomades and muds are lighter and tend to offer softer, more natural results.

Alterna Hemp Seed Sculpting Putty (Wax)
Alterna Hemp Styling Mud (Pomade)
American Crew Pomade
Bumble and Bumble Styling Wax
CHI Matte Wax
Kenra Platinum Texturizing Taffy
Kenra Platinum Working Wax
Sebastian Molding Mud

Heat Protectants

WHEN TO USE: As needed. Heat protectants are a must if you'll be styling your hair with blow dryers, flatirons, curling irons, and other heat appliances. They are also great for protecting against sun damage and humidity. You'll find these products in virtually every form imaginable, from sprays and serums to creams and gels. The best heat protection comes from silicone-based products because they create a strong barrier between your hair and the heat. If your hair is fine or is easily weighed down, go for spray or mist-type products. For medium-coarse or thick hair, serums are your best bet.

BioSilk Silk Therapy
CHI Silk Infusion
CHI 44 Iron Guard Thermal Protection
    Spray
FHI Heat Hot Sauce
got2b Guardian Angel Heat Protect N' Blow
    Out Lotion and Gloss Finish
John Frieda Frizz-Ease Thermal Protection
    Hair Serum
Kenra Straightening Serum
Nexxus Heat Protexx
Redken Smooth Down Heat Glide Smoother
Sedu Anti-Frizz Polishing Treatment with
    Argan Oil
Tigi S-Factor Heat Defender Flat Iron Shine
    Spray
Wella Professionals Dry Thermal Image Spray

Setting Lotions/Design Foams

WHEN TO USE: As needed. These products help mold and set wet hair.

Design Essentials Compositions Foaming
    Wrap Lotion
Giovanni Sculpting/Setting Lotion
Lottabody Texturizing Hair Setting Lotion
Jane Carter Solution Wrap and Roll
KeraCare Foam Wrap
Mizani Setting Lotion

Serums and Shine Sprays

WHEN TO USE: As needed. These products add incredible shine and polish to your finished style. Some of these products can also be used for heat protection.

Biosilk Silk Therapy
Citre Shine Color Prism Anti Frizz Serum
L'ANZA Healing Strength Neem Plant Silk
    Serum
Kenra Platinum Silkening Gloss
Paul Mitchell Super Skinny Serum
Oscar Blandi Olio Di Jasmine Shine Spray
Pureology Shine Max- Shining Hair Smoother

Hair Sprays (Aerosol)

WHEN TO USE: As needed. These products are great for finishing and setting a style on fine- to medium-textured hair without weighing it down.

Back to Basics Firm Hold Hair Spray
Kenra Volume Spray
Sebastian Shaper PLUS
Scruples High Definition Firm Shaping Spray
TIGI Bed Head Hard Head Hairspray

Index

W

20447765R10148